NO LONGER PROPERTY OF
SEATTLE PUBLIC LIBRARY

RECEIVED
NOV   2019
By

ARE MEN
ANIMALS?

ARE MEN ANIMALS?

HOW MODERN MASCULINITY SELLS MEN SHORT

MATTHEW GUTMANN

BASIC BOOKS

New York

Copyright © 2019 by Matthew Gutmann
Cover design by Rodrigo Corral
Cover image © Pakorn Kumruen / EyeEm
Cover copyright © 2019 Hachette Book Group, Inc.

Hachette Book Group supports the right to free expression and the value of copyright. The purpose of copyright is to encourage writers and artists to produce the creative works that enrich our culture.

The scanning, uploading, and distribution of this book without permission is a theft of the author's intellectual property. If you would like permission to use material from the book (other than for review purposes), please contact permissions@hbgusa.com. Thank you for your support of the author's rights.

Basic Books
Hachette Book Group
1290 Avenue of the Americas, New York, NY 10104
www.basicbooks.com
Printed in the United States of America
First Edition: November 2019
Published by Basic Books, an imprint of Perseus Books, LLC, a subsidiary of Hachette Book Group, Inc. The Basic Books name and logo is a trademark of the Hachette Book Group.

The Hachette Speakers Bureau provides a wide range of authors for speaking events. To find out more, go to www.hachettespeakersbureau.com or call (866) 376-6591.

The publisher is not responsible for websites (or their content) that are not owned by the publisher.

Print book interior design by Linda Mark.

Library of Congress Cataloging-in-Publication Data
Names: Gutmann, Matthew C., 1953– author.
Title: Are men animals? : how modern masculinity sells men short / Matthew Gutmann.
Description: First edition. | New York : Basic Books, [2019] | Includes bibliographical references and index.
Identifiers: LCCN 2019014412 (print) | LCCN 2019016525 (ebook) | ISBN 9781541699595 (ebook) | ISBN 9781541699588 (hardcover)
Subjects: LCSH: Masculinity. | Sex role. | Men–Identity.
Classification: LCC BF692.5 (ebook) | LCC BF692.5 .G88 2019 (print) | DDC 155.3/32–dc23
LC record available at https://lccn.loc.gov/2019014412

ISBNs: 978-1-5416-9958-8 (hardcover), 978-1-5416-9959-5 (ebook)

LSC-C

10 9 8 7 6 5 4 3 2 1

To my brothers, Rob and Rick

Ain't we both members of de same club—de Hairy Apes?

Yank, in *The Hairy Ape*, EUGENE O'NEILL

CONTENTS

INTRODUCTION

W<small>E PLACE UNREASONABLE TRUST IN BIOLOGICAL EXPLANATIONS</small> of male behavior. In early 2018, for example, *Newsweek* carried a story titled "Men Who Like Jazz Have Less Testosterone Than Those Who Like Rock." It was an eye-catching headline. Although it relied on ideas we may already have about gender and behavior, it was meant to tease us with a fun bit of new information. Perhaps some readers were ready to accept the conclusion that rock 'n' roll was manlier, because they thought this musical genre was more nakedly belligerent, and testosterone was a hormone they associated with aggressive masculinity.

Other readers might have been pleased by the Japanese study on which the article reported, because it made a correlation between high intelligence and the preference for what the authors considered "sophisticated music"—classical, jazz, and world music. But even for the readers who agreed with the conclusion that hard rockers must have more testosterone, there was just one little problem: it was absolute nonsense. The study was based on a minuscule sampling of men. Just how many men had been included in the study they claimed proved a connection between "rebellious music such as hard rock" and higher levels of testosterone? A grand total of thirty-seven, all young male students in Japan from universities and vocational schools.

These thirty-seven Japanese students were thus asked to stand in for the males of the world, all times and all places, as to the links between their "endocrinological predispositions and patterns of music preference." The study contained zero cultural analysis about who was listening to rock, classical, and jazz music in Japan. Old or young? Urban or rural? Highly educated? People who had traveled abroad? It could all be explained by endocrinology, so why bother with demography? All it took for *Newsweek* to run with the story was the discovery of a claim made in a scientific journal that fit a preconception about manliness.[1]

This sort of conclusion is all too common. There is a pull on scientists hungry for funding that can lead some to play fast and loose when it comes to research about all kinds of sexy topics, from the effects of caffeine to mind reading to, well, sex. Journalists covering the sciences can feel similarly pressured to embellish the facts based on what they perceive will go over well with their readers. Yet researching the connection between biology and behavior can be dangerous. When journalists jump at the newest alleged association between a biological factor and human behavior, we often gain more insight into preexisting cultural prejudices than into new scientific discoveries. You like rock music? You obviously have a higher level of testosterone, which, as we all know, means you are more of a man. You like jazz? You might be more sophisticated, but you are also less manly.

Uncritical deference to biological explanations of behavior infects our thinking about women as well as men, but in recent decades, women have done a better job pushing back. Most people now understand, for example, that there is no predictable correlation between women's menstrual cycles and their moods. But boys will still be boys, right? Despite decades of research contradicting this conclusion, we are still completely willing to believe that men can best be understood by looking more closely at their brains, balls, and biceps.[2]

Every day people are confronted with biological terms relating to hormones, genes, heredity, and evolution as they try to comprehend male sexuality and violence, as if these biological clues explain what makes men behave the way they do. One particularly effective strategy is to compare the males of the human variety with males of other animal species. When we do this, we tend to simplify the behavior of men to emphasize automatic, animalistic responses to stimuli. There is no room for the enormous range of male responses based on culture, history, and personality, and therefore no need for accountability. (And, let's admit it, that is not being fair to nonhuman males, either.) If we hold that human male behavior is best understood in relation to what the males of diverse species do and feel, driven by instinct and impulse, then we are indeed selling men short. Men are animals. But what does that really mean?

Few people are so blind as to think that biology determines everything about what it means to be a man. But how many of us can claim not to harbor more than a sneaking suspicion that men's physiology explains a lot of their behavior? It is difficult to resist the tidiness of biological answers to life's big questions. Witness the popularity of the genealogy companies 23andMe and Ancestry.com, which make millions of dollars by indulging people's beliefs that their DNA tells them "who they are," and that their personality and character are somehow rooted in their ancestry.

How we talk about men, even in a casual or offhanded way, determines what we expect of men. Take testosterone. Some of our most widely read and smartest pundits casually endow this molecule with supernatural properties to make broader points about men. A search of daily news sources quickly yields mentions like: "a cloud of testosterone" (Frank Bruni), "hard-driving testosterone-fueled culture" (Walter Isaacson), "rhetorical-testosterone deficit" (Kathleen Parker), "testosterone-drenched" movie stars (in an article on an up-and-coming young actor), and "testosterone-measuring handshakes" (Charles Blow). James Lee Burke, one of my favorite mystery writers, leaves an indelible image in a 2016 novel: "I could hear him breathing and could smell the testosterone that seemed ironed into his clothes."[3]

It's not hard to see the poetic license here. But the pattern is meaningful because using testosterone as a figure of speech to describe masculinity has become harmful. When we view aggressive handshakes as explained by chemicals we are asking for trouble. And the tacit assumptions behind this way of talking are continually reinforced by poorly designed or misinterpreted research that lets men off the hook when they misbehave by attributing their behavior to distinctive male traits. Biology seems fixed. So by gluing it to male behavior, men can be exonerated for acts associated with male excess, particularly sexual violence. To the extent we believe in biobabble about men and their behavior, we naturalize patriarchal relationships themselves.[4]

What people believe about the intrinsic, natural characteristics of men has direct implications as much for political process as for our interpersonal relations, sometimes in related ways. A young man came up to me after a lecture I gave in the fall of 2017. He told me, "My mother voted for Trump. I think she overlooked his comments about women, because, you know, 'Boys will be boys.'" The student paused, looking sheepish as he continued, "What I want to ask her, though, is 'Is that what you think of *me*?'" He was clearly in distress imagining that his mother could lump him together with Donald Trump just because they both were men. "Did you talk to your mother about this, about how you feel?" I asked. He responded with the saddest face and said, "I can't ask her. I'm scared to know the answer."

I will get to Trump and the widespread acquiescence to his misogyny in due course. For now, he can serve as the archetype of seemingly intransigent beliefs about men's inherent proclivities, including the extent to which people have come to believe that men's biology regulates their sexuality and aggression, that only fools try to deny these truths, and that societies must be structured to accommodate and constrain them.

Male-or-female categories persist for all sorts of reasons, both practical and obsolete. When we watch Animal Planet, available on televisions in seventy countries worldwide, we nod with approval when we learn, "The male swan helps build the nest, while the female swan incubates the eggs." This division of labor aligns with our ideas about the division of human labor. And exceptions to male-female swan behavior are not found. So it is remarkably easy to make the cognitive leap to thinking, "Well, maybe the human male-female patterns I am familiar with are hard-and-fast, too. Maybe my husband can't really change."

Biological extremism about men and boys is nonsense. But it's nonsense with a tenacious hold on our imaginations, seemingly rooted in our experience and scientific evidence. Speaking about the influence of biological determinants of behavior, the eminent neuroscientist Robert Sapolsky once asked, "Why are people such suckers for the idea that genes are the be-all and end-all? It's particularly bad right now." He went on to refute the bad science behind such ideas but left the social roots of the predilection dangling.[5]

Men's biology hasn't substantially changed in tens of thousands of years. And for this reason alone the crisis in masculinity we face today can't be understood or combated through a narrow biological lens. That's where this book comes in. As an anthropologist, I use a different set of tools to answer the question about why people are such suckers for "Boys will be boys"—and why too many scientists are accomplices. Anthropology can uncover the complicated cultural origins of seemingly biological male behavior and show how certain essentialized beliefs about maleness promoted by scientists are themselves products of the same cultural influences. Scientists can be just as susceptible as nonprofessionals to thinking that particular chromosomes and hormones reveal the secret codes of human maleness, that there is just something about being a man.

I believe that the ways in which people think about men and expect men to behave can be dramatically renegotiated, but that this will require us to understand the entrenched views about men and women that we're up against. And make no mistake: assumptions about male biological natures are just as intricately woven into the fabric of well-educated and liberal sectors of society as they are in conservative communities. How these wrongheaded ideas about maleness are expressed varies from place to place around the globe, but a startling feature of the contemporary world is how normal it is to hear people couch ideas about men, sexuality, and aggression in the language of pseudoscience.

An example: unchallenged assumptions about men's underlying sexual and aggressive nature have received flagrant expression in the practice of modern militaries to ensure that male soldiers have access to sex with women and that they have adequate and regular release for their "sexual energies." The French army has called them *bordels militaires de campagne*, and they proliferated in World Wars I and II and the wars in Indochina and Algeria. Never to be outdone, in one notorious example, on August 23, 1945, the US military authorities in charge of the occupation of Japan decided to set up a Recreation and Amusement Association, press-ganging 55,000 women to provide sexual services for the occupying troops. Official rest and recreation (R&R) centers sponsored barely disguised brothels for US soldiers during the Vietnam War.

In one of his novels, Mario Vargas Llosa has a military general complain, on behalf of male soldiers isolated in the Peruvian jungle, that "in short, abstinence makes for a hell of a lot of corruption. And demoralization, nervousness, apathy." If you agree that men more than women have a particular and inveterate necessity for regular sexual release, then this all might make sense. But recognize the stakes here. Are you really ready to cede operating rights over men's bodies to impulses that men themselves cannot be expected to control?[6]

There are practical implications if you think men's bodies control their destiny, because it will affect how you understand basic matters like nurturance, ambition, competitiveness, forgiveness, assault, and war. Underlying beliefs about male sexuality can give scientific-sounding credence to claims that men's and women's sex drives are by nature distinct, and these claims in turn can help to explain why no new birth control methods have been developed for men in centuries, and why it might seem to make sense that so often birth control arbitrarily remains a woman's responsibility.

Why biological explanations are so widespread, popular, and persuasive, and why biology has become a catchall explanatory tool today for understanding men, is not primarily a result of new scientific findings about testosterone, the cerebral cortex, or DNA. After all, the research doesn't actually provide persuasive answers to the questions being asked. If the general public has become overly dependent on explanations patchworked together from gene interactions, hormone levels, and primate cousins, then it's time to ask why this trend is happening now and why it's been growing over recent decades.

One key to undoing these taken-for-granted ideas about maleness is to study the actual diversity of men and masculinities across time and place. Believing that your own experience as a man or with men is pretty much the way it is for everyone else, everywhere else, might seem reasonable, but in fact, as we will see, it is mistaken. Most importantly, there is more in jeopardy than right and wrong ideas: subliminal concepts about men as some kind of timeless and cultureless species apart feed into the thinking, "Don't blame me. I'm a guy!" Nonsense.

Acting as if men can't control themselves is hazardous. Naming a problem is an important part of solving it. So, here's the issue as I see it: not only do we reach too quickly for biological explanations of male sexuality and violence, terrain not firm enough to support our conclusions, but the very language we employ about men compounds the problems by fossilizing masculinity and maleness. Because men are not a chain of chromosomal clones, by exploring the roots of the attraction to rigid biological explanations about men and their so-called inborn characteristics, we can free ourselves of unnecessary, self-imposed restrictions in how we think about male behavior.

Also unacknowledged is the fact that, for most men in the world, most of the time, women are central to what it means to be a man. Being a man first and foremost for most men means not being a woman. To be sure, there are other ways men define themselves and are defined: feeling more or less manly in comparison to other men, feeling more or less manly than other men at particular times, not being another kind of man (thin, rich, straight, hairy, white). Yet just as it is mistaken to think that men's biology dictates that they have too little control over themselves, it is dangerous not to see women as central to everything about men, too.

There has certainly been a tendency in discussions of men and masculinity to assume that male-only interactions and spaces imply that women are largely irrelevant to men, at least after they reach adulthood. No one could deny the importance of women in the lives of children, starting with mothers. But it has been harder to think about the influence of women on men.

To say women are central to everything in the lives of men is more than a matter of mothers spending more time raising sons than fathers do with daughters, although that is important, as is the fact that mothers are routinely more present role models for daughters than fathers are with sons. We need to understand the influence women have not only on boys but also on adult males. We need to understand that women are central to most men's very sense of manliness and virility. This means paying attention to the opinions and experiences of women regarding men, and how, for many men, masculinities develop and transform and have little meaning except in relation to women and female identities and activities in all their similar diversity and complexity.

This book is more about men than women, in order to focus the study and because there are specific problems that need our special attention. But women are relevant to many aspects of men's lives, including when they are not physically present; their interpretation of events, identities, and activities involving men could not be more fundamental in making sense of men's control over their own beliefs and actions.

So throughout the book I use examples from the lives of women as well as men to understand modern men and masculinities. There is also a lot we can learn from decades of studies about women. After all, women are animals, too, and women have historically been the target of mountains of biobabble asserting that their bodies yoke them to one or another lowly behavior.

Where does masculinity come from? We need to address the idea, often taken as irrefutable fact, that male behavior is essentially identical across human history and the animal kingdom. Consider, for example, the following myths and half-myths:

- *With few exceptions, males spend less time and energy in parental activities than females.* One, there are important counterexamples among humans as well as among nonhuman animals. Two, and more importantly, among humans we see enormous "elasticity," that is, malleability and variation in patterns of parenting behavior—an ability among men to do "women's work" and vice versa. For example, when women migrate for work, men can and do take on far more parenting duties than we typically expect of them.
- *Despite fervent and noble efforts, anthropologists have been unable to locate a matriarchal social structure anywhere on earth.* True, but what does this actually tell us? In another example of elasticity, for the first time ever, in the past one hundred years of human history we have seen women rise to become political leaders in almost every country on earth. We are nowhere near equity, but pointing in that direction.
- *Except in the movies, we always find more men than women in the military.* There are no longer physical reasons for this imbalance; culture, not biology, explains the disparity, even if Amazons have never existed except in Seattle.[7]

- *In culture after culture, sexual humor features more male than female exploits and fantasies.* This is not an unsurprising finding if the people collecting and recounting sexual humor are men. Here and elsewhere, we should not make so many assumptions about female sexuality if we are just talking to men about men.
- *Troops of chimpanzees, "our closest cousins," are led by alpha males, not females.* It turns out that another of "our closest cousins," bonobos, are alpha-female led.

The problem with every example here is that each one only superficially supports the claim, the supposedly irrefutable fact, that male behavior is consistent across human history and the animal kingdom. It is not consistent at all, in reality, and the first thing we need to do is pluralize. Instead of masculinity, we should think masculini*ties*. Far from being irrefutable facts, many of our assumptions about men and masculinity are based on cultural beliefs dressed up in biological clothing. The phrase "Boys will be boys" carries with it the implicit notion that men are born and not made, and that as a result there is little that parents and societies can do to influence their desires and behaviors — we can't fight biology; it's better to focus on ways to restrain them and their diehard impulses.

And why is it that we use the phrase "Boys will be boys" only when we are saying something negative about what boys or men do? Somehow when men and boys do something thoughtful and generous we don't hear anyone maintain, "Well, you know, he did really well cleaning up his room because, after all, boys will be boys." Biology governs the rules of male misbehavior; only individual male exceptions to the rule can explain when they do something positive.[8]

In the United States we say "Boys will be boys." In Mexico we say "Así son" ([That's] the way they are), meaning that's the way men are. The meanings of "manly" in modern China have fluctuated from the zealous Red Guard to the "search for the ideal man" to the wily capitalist entrepreneur who knows you need to quote science to be considered enlightened and successful. And though it doesn't apply just to men, there is a Chinese saying, "You can't stop a dog from eating shit," that is often applied to boys; it means that we just have to accept that that's the way they are and they are never going to change.[9]

In France you sometimes hear "Ça, c'est bien les hommes" (That's men for you). In Portuguese, the relevant saying is "Como um rapaz" (Just like a boy). According to classicists, the expression "Boys will be boys" can be traced all the way back to an ancient Roman proverb: "Sunt pueri pueri, pueri puerilia tractant" (Boys are boys, and boys will act like boys). I do like how Latin hammers home the point about puerility.

Language matters, and the half-joke about the English expression "Boys will be boys" is no longer funny.

Among the delights and difficulties of studying gender and sexuality is that literally everyone has experiences and opinions about them. And questions. And disagreements. Through examples drawn from the anthropological treasure chest, and some personal anecdotes, this book will provide insights for our daily discussions about what men are like deep down, what we can reasonably expect from men, and what we should expect from ourselves *as* men. When teens undergo a circumcision rite among the Gisu in Uganda, they aim to tame "the wild animal," so they can gain self-control and become responsible adult men. Historians of Europe write in the same vein that mastering one's sexual drives has long been considered a sign of mental health and credibility, with lack of manly control indicating mental illness. In some historical periods, women's supposed lack of such control was taken as evidence that they could not be trusted with important decisions or leadership roles. Of course, when the script flipped—supposing men's unruly libidos to be higher—that became evidence that women's delicate and demure constitutions must be kept well away from the sexually charged male atmospheres of politics and commerce.[10]

There has always been talk about men, and men writing about men, in every social commentary down through the ages. The difference now is that we are thinking about and discussing, positively and negatively,

men as gendered, too. Although the term "gender" (as in gender issues, gender rights, gender equality) is often synonymous with "women"
(women's issues, women's rights, women's equality), it should not be.
Gender applies, and should apply, to men as much as women. Anthropologists have long debated what exactly this might mean. Some studies
in the 1970s suggested there were widespread global and historical patterns associating men with culture and women with nature, men with
public spaces and women with private ones. Since then, feminists and
other scholars have continued to grapple with whether we can reasonably make these and other cross-cultural generalizations about men,
maleness, and masculinities.

We know that biology matters, and sexual reproduction is a clear
illustration of important physiological differences between women
and men. The fact that only women get pregnant and lactate is of obvious and fundamental significance and basic to a variety of gendered
divisions of labor that have always been central features of human
existence. The rub has come when we extrapolated from these real
biological differences between men and women to assume that we
could also explain other differences as biologically rooted in sex—
for example, leadership ability, aptitude for mathematics, capacity for
nurturing, logical reasoning, or intelligence.

The twentieth century proved to be a turning point in uncovering
the extent to which apparent gender differences were not truly biological. The widespread introduction of reliable contraceptives (and plum-
meting fertility rates), improvements in obstetrics and women's health
in general (and reduced rates of maternal and infant mortality), commercial baby formula, and powerful feminist political movements have
unmistakably transformed gendered divisions of labor in every corner of
the globe. Or, better put, they have provided conditions in which these
divisions of labor could change.

Despite these changes, ideas about men's and women's involuntary
natures persist, to such a degree that we badly need to look more closely
at what, after all, is biological, and less amenable to change, and where

our own blinkered preconceptions about biology and sex have limited our expectations. Compared to the beginning of the twentieth century, many more people now know how hideous and horrific it is to believe that certain races are naturally more or less intelligent, industrious, or hypersexual. We need a similar challenge to our understanding of maleness and femaleness, our language about these issues, and the attributes commonly considered intrinsic to one or the other.

In these pages, we will go from Mexico City to Shanghai, from rehab programs in Oakland to the frontlines of war in Iraq, from the tragedy of sexual exploitation and abuse among UN peacekeepers in Haiti to the seemingly nonpartisan laboratories of endocrinologists. Thoughtful dialogue on these matters has never been more important, after the most publicized and consequential sex crimes in the history of the United States swept the country in 2017 and 2018. At the heart of every one of them was the question of men's sexuality, how standardized it is, whether boys and men learn to act out their sexualities in certain ways, and whether they can be rehabilitated when things go seriously awry. Here, we will address the basic concerns running through each new revelation: Is there something inherent in men that makes them more prone to committing sexual assault? Are all men like this, or just some of those with power? Do they rape and murder because that's what the males of the species do—indeed, is this what they all would do, if they thought they could get away with it?

We need to learn to better distinguish folk beliefs from underlying biological compulsions and restraints. Although I will not dismiss genes, hormones, and evolution, I will indicate when biological explanations reach beyond their reasonable limits. It's long past time for the social sciences to work more closely with the life sciences and to get beyond biology-as-strawman for humanist ridicule.

This book is also about global cultural responses to the problems of misogyny and male violence. The powerful #MeToo movement that swept through the United States in 2017 demanded that men's sexual assaults on women stop. Activists spent less time wondering why men

were doing these things in the first place. Was it hard-wiring? Their evolutionary drives? Even those who work tirelessly for gender equality are
affected by widespread theories about men's fixed temperament. Some
people insist that gender categories like "man" and "woman" are irrelevant to our daily interactions. Others strongly oppose any departure
from two-gender thinking.

Anthropologists study patterns of human existence. We ask philosophical questions about what it means to be human, and our answers
consider what happens not just between birth and death, but between
conception and funeral. We look for commonalities but thrive on variation, because this proves how many options are available to us. That
is why my approach in this study is to cast the net as widely as I can,
which because of my own research experience means especially over
the United States, Mexico, and China, to demonstrate regularities
and anomalies, ambiguities and certitudes, when it comes to men and
masculinities in the twenty-first century. The wave of retrenched conservative gender relations may take different forms in different places,
but it is unmistakably global. More than just describing my observations and conversations with men and women about men, I hope to
make clear both that this means the stakes are especially high and
urgent and that the opportunities are great.

This will be a collective effort. If you are complacent about wage gaps
or the lack of child care, you are part of the problem. If you raise your children by selectively warning the boys not to pressure the girls for sex, and
the girls to be careful around the boys when it comes to sex, you are part
of the problem. If you never question why all the modern forms of contraception are designed for women, or why only young men have to register
for the draft, you are part of the problem. Maybe you, too, maintain some
less examined, undeclared notions about men's and women's natures and
conduct your life with at least implicitly naturalized gender guidelines.

Such confusing times provide openings for change that we can't
afford to miss.

CHAPTER ONE

GENDER CONFUSION

We're living in transitional times.

LAURA KIPNIS

A SPECTER IS HAUNTING THE WORLD—THE SPECTER OF GENDER confusion. It plays out in the tug-of-war between conservative and progressive understandings of gender, of maleness and femaleness and other kinds of genderness. Gender-benders embrace the specter, while fundamentalists attempt exorcisms. All around us, gender confusion incites furious debate and anguished questioning. It offers a good opportunity to take stock of men, to reassess and renegotiate what maleness means, and to examine why our beliefs about biology and masculinity seem to map so neatly onto our social and political credos. We need to be clearer about gender confusion, better at distinguishing anxieties and limitations from expectations and choices, more determined than ever to untangle the fairy tales about men from the bodies and souls of real live men.

Admittedly, gender confusion is a developing phenomenon. We still ask, "Is it a boy or a girl?" But even basic ways of defining gender can easily confound us now. Boy or girl? And later, straight or gay or gender nonconforming? Even distinguishing between "sex" and "gender"—how

15

they are both different and intertwined—has become a constant source of reflection and disagreement. Signaling widespread debate and confusion over gender issues, sociologist Michael Kimmel helped launch contemporary feminist studies of men and masculinities with a provocation: "This, then, is the great secret of American manhood: *We are afraid of other men*. Homophobia is a central organizing principle of our cultural definition of manhood."[1]

WHAT'S CONFUSING?

When gay marriage was legalized in Mexico City in late 2009 (almost six years before it happened for the United States at the federal level), it represented a sea change in attitudes about men and their sexuality—as well as, of course, women and their sexuality. In households around the country arguments erupted about men, love, sex, parenting, religion, and progress.

When mass murderers in the United States are time and again young, white, and male, we are not certain if the link between maleness and violence should be a central part of the deliberations about causes and solutions.

When women and children are offered separate cars on urban subways around the world, we all know this measure is to protect women from men, but uncertainty remains about whether sexual assaults are acts we can stop or just interrupt.

When transgender politics are front and center on popular television programs, and answers to questions about "gender" on application forms can no longer be contained in neat pairs of two, what makes someone a man is increasingly up for grabs. On college campuses, students meeting for the first time now routinely share their names, years, majors, and preferred pronouns: suddenly and seemingly out of nowhere, he/she is too antiquated and restrictive for a younger generation.

As women in the United States recovered after the 2008 Great Recession, landing more jobs more quickly than men, men's contributions to families and communities got reexamined, and the image of man-the-breadwinner became blurrier.

When women who are unmarried by a certain age in China are publicly shamed, people reasonably ask whether men should be treated the same way and why they are not.

When a woman is gang raped on a moving bus in Delhi, or Muslim women are similarly assaulted by Christian Serbs in Bosnia, or when young women in the United States are sexually attacked by young men on college campuses, we ask why. Maybe we say the men are behaving like most male animals do when they can. When confronted by examples like these, often we ask if there isn't something basic to maleness that compels men as a category to assault women, especially under certain conditions.

All this leads to confusion, debate, concern, and turmoil. Elementary school children come home for supper and ask what a sex change operation is, and can they have one. Debates unfurl about changing titles from Miss and Mrs. to Ms., and then Ms. and Mr. to Mx. Stores carry "gender-neutral clothing." Revisions from one edition to another of the *Diagnostic and Statistical Manual of Mental Disorders* become fodder for arguments among a remarkably broad swath of the population about which gender identities are "normal." Segregated bathrooms, previously spaces generating little controversy, suddenly become the sites of moral panic and legal battles.

After years of debate, gay marriage and gays in the US military receive state sanction. That might feel like a certain resolution to gender confusion. But before anyone could catch their breath, the US Supreme Court informed the world that gays could not receive the same protections as straights (from cake makers, for example), and the president of the United States announced that transgender men and women were officially unwelcome in the US armed forces after all.[2]

For many LGBTQ activists and scholars in the United States and elsewhere, discrimination against trans people is projected as the next major domain of erotic life to be questioned. Trans politics has captured the popular imagination, triggered new kinds of gender confusion, and highlighted the ties between life, love, and work. As an indication of just how much has changed in a short period of time, consider that in 1996 I was interviewed for a job that was to be a joint appointment between anthropology and gender studies, and at the end of my interview for the position, the chair of the search committee asked me, "Would you consider a sex change operation?" I would like to think that as a result of significant changes in social mores around transsexuality, no one could get away with such a jest twenty years later.

Some elements of gender confusion arise from new conditions, and some aspects of gender have always been more complicated than we may have acknowledged. In recent decades, in the United States and throughout the world, the number of women attending universities has surpassed the number of men. The long-term implications of this trend are only just becoming apparent, including employment patterns, wage differentials, and property ownership. The sudden emergence of the #MeToo movement has demanded an end to male sexual harassment and assault and galvanized women across generations, while men in fields from filmmaking to journalism to academia have fallen from positions of authority.

At the same time, some of our confusion about gender stems from superficial thinking in the past. If gender is often invoked as a way to highlight social problems such as bias and abuse against women by men, how can the same term apply just as much to men as women? After all, men don't generally face the same kinds of gender discrimination or harassment. The reason is that when we note that men have gender it just means we need to stop treating men as the default human, what sociolinguists call the unmarked category, the group that is the stand-in for everyone. We assume so much about men that goes unspecified, or unremarked, as if only women have gender. Despite this failing, both men and women are products of social norms and expectations related to gender; neither is sprung ready-made simply because of the configuration of the body.[3]

Our tacit beliefs about unmarked male behavior often color our reactions to male misbehavior, from the criminal to the mundane. This is true as a general rule, but that rule can be challenged, especially at pivotal moments in history. Feminist scholar Gayle Rubin's insights are particularly relevant to understanding what is at stake in reassessing men and masculinities today. In a 1984 essay, she argued that "contemporary conflicts over sexual values and erotic conduct have much in common with the religious disputes of earlier centuries." By comparing sexual and religious claims, Rubin sought to elevate sexual politics in the historical record as deserving of recognition and reexamination.

Even more, taking advantage of the widespread understanding that there were defining moments in the history of religious beliefs and practices, Rubin showed that the same could be said for the history of sexuality. By documenting that there are some "historical periods in which sexuality is more sharply contested and more overtly politicized" than in others, she concluded that in these moments, "the domain of erotic life is, in effect, renegotiated." In other words, during periods of broad social stress, attitudes about sexuality that may have been accepted for centuries can begin to collapse and change.[4]

Gender is not the same thing as sex or sexuality. These terms are notoriously difficult to define, but at the risk of oversimplifying, let's say that usually sex relates to certain biological matters, while gender concerns certain social matters. Sexuality's biological matters are in turn tough to define. Are these always related to reproduction, for example? Not really, because reproduction doesn't cover oral sex. Regardless, Rubin's points about sexuality apply to gender, too, because in certain moments in history we find heightened tension and confusion around gender, and it is precisely at those moments that change can occur, particularly change concerning what we take for granted about gender. Take the military, for example, which often offers illustrations of changing social mores about women and men. When recruitment into the US armed forces seriously lagged in the 1970s, suddenly women were called in to fill the ranks. Attitudes about women and about military service had to change.

There is a caveat, however, in that how things change, and in what direction, is never preordained. It is not inconceivable that if at some future date the military was again able to fill its rolls with men alone, a "reassessment" could be made, declaring that women were again by nature unfit or less fit than men for military assignments, including those involving combat. Call it the Handmaid's Tale Cautionary Principle: the contest over the future of gender will be determined by the people who live it, so presume nothing for sure about what comes next. People advocating either retrenched conservatism or progressive change are at this very moment vying to resolve gender confusion in one direction or another. Central to the struggle to reassess and renegotiate maleness and masculinities is what we make of men and their bodies.

The Handmaid's Tale scenario can be alarming, because it is not too far-fetched to imagine that there are men who would advocate for the enslavement of women for their own pleasure. Think "incels," young men who believe they are "involuntarily celibate," and that women are torturing them by refusing to have sex with them. Many conservatives acknowledge that women have changed what they expect of men in recent decades, but their aversion to gender change has a fatal flaw: it leaves men behind. With the simplistic reasoning that men are just naturally the way they are, these conservatives leave no room for the possibility of male change: in terms of educational and career achievements, for example, they fear that men will never again outshine women, who for their part over the past century have made significant progress toward gender equality and show no signs of ceding this ground. Women will not suddenly acquiesce to sexual assaults. They will not retreat en masse from working outside their homes. They will not give up their positions of power in business, education, the arts, or government to return to the all-male days. Nor will they give up the vote. And why should they? These gains are hard-won and are now part of our culture. So where does this leave men? That's a big part of what this book aims to address. If past notions of masculinity are no longer working for many women, men themselves need to explore their options. As often as not, the stimulus to change is coming from women, but the resolution, by definition, must involve men as key players. From confusion, resentment, and even anger can come transformation.[5]

Women are challenging men to change. They are catalysts for gender change overall. But in order to understand what can and should be expected of men, we first need to understand what men are and can be. There is more involved than men doing their share of domestic work, as important as that is. There are lives on the line. For many around the world, this era of gender instability is a confusing and precarious time. But it is also potentially a time of awakening.

GENDER CONFUSION NOW

How much biology is held responsible for any human attribute, like race or maleness, is conditioned by the social and political landscape in particular periods of time. The assumptions we make about reflexive qualities associated with men and masculinities are also directly shaped by how much we know about men in diverse cultural settings and historical periods quite different from our own.

For much of the twentieth century in the United States, our dialogue on the relationship between biology and gender has been never ending. Scientific racism and its corollaries under eugenics, as well as scientific sexism, taken for granted in the 1910s and 1920s, came under withering attack in the heyday of social unrest in the 1930s, when progressive ideas about practically everything permeated the social fabric. Post–World War II conservatism tried to reestablish women's intrinsic place in the kitchen and home, but it was then broadly opposed in the upheavals of the 1960s and early 1970s. A backlash against feminism followed, taking scientific form in the mid-1970s with the proclamation of an all-encompassing sociobiological theory, which exerted tremendous influence in one form or another in subsequent decades. Never without controversy, the Human Genome Project of the 1990s represented, after eugenics, the second major push of the century for what Jonathan Marks calls "hereditarian scientific ideology." The #MeToo movement of the late 2010s, though not often directly addressing the issue of what is incorrigible in men, heralded a major counteroffensive against the norms of male sexual predation.[6]

The trend that emerges from this history is that science often amplifies discourse more than it changes it. Science conveys legitimacy on prevailing ideas (for example, about gender) that themselves arise from political viewpoints. Writing about social Darwinism in the early twentieth century, historian Richard Hofstadter noted, "In determining whether such ideas are accepted, truth and logic are less important criteria than suitability to the intellectual needs and preconceptions of social interests." To determine the truth and logic of ideas about men and maleness, it never hurts to consider whose interests are served by which viewpoints.[7]

Dominant theories on human nature—especially racialized and sexualized human natures—had already passed through wild swings in the twentieth century. Scientists had alternated between two poles: one emphasizing that it was physiology that determined aptitude, interests, and abilities, and another stressing instead the role of social constraints and opportunities in the expression of our humanity. In periods of significant social ferment, including around gender issues—for example, the 1930s, 1960s, and 2010s in the United States—gender confusion has prevailed, often in dialogue with influential scientific and public opinion about men and women and whether they are meaningfully dissimilar by nature.

In her history of how aggression and animality became inextricably linked in "colloquial science" in the post–World War II United States, for example, Erika Lorraine Milam asks, "How did evolutionists become trusted experts on questions of humanity's fundamental essence?" She describes a shift away from comparing life to machines: "Evolutionists imagined human nature as continuous with animal behavior," and thus "evolutionary theory could speak to a more fundamental question—what did it mean to be human?" Evolutionists, geneticists, and endocrinologists today share the rights to scientifically explain maleness. What these approaches all share is the notion of the body at the center of their scientific definitions of humanness.[8]

In a sense, you could say that 1949 was a turning point in modern debates about whether we are prisoners of our bodies. That year, French philosopher Simone de Beauvoir published her luminous manifesto *The Second Sex*. In it, she critiqued assumptions about intrinsic female behavior and the female body, famously writing that biological considerations "are one of the keys to the understanding of woman. But I deny that they establish for her a fixed and inevitable destiny. They are insufficient for setting up a hierarchy of the sexes; they fail to explain why woman is the Other; they do not condemn her to remain in this subordinate role forever." *The Second Sex* was a foundational text for feminist movements across the globe, in part because it defied the widely held idea that women's bodies uniquely constrained their abilities and actions.[9]

But *The Second Sex* became a foundational text not in the decade of the 1950s after it was published, but only later, in the 1960s, as part of the political upsurge challenging male domination and all that came with it. The book contributed to that upsurge, but it needed a political movement to achieve its fuller impact.

By the time de Beauvoir's study appeared, shortly after World War II, tensions between support for women's fuller economic participation mixed uneasily with a set of retrenched conservative cultural restrictions on women. It was another time of heightened gender confusion and contestation. By the 1960s, inspired in the United States and elsewhere by the civil rights movement, and later, the anti–Vietnam War movement, the feminist wave rose to new heights.

Not everyone was happy with feminism. Notable in the backlash against radical social change was a landmark publication in 1975 titled *Sociobiology: The New Synthesis*, by Edward O. Wilson. In this text,

Wilson explained the social behavior of humans and other animals as functions of biological evolution, offering a macroscopic view in which "the humanities and social sciences shrink to specialized branches of biology." Wilson, the chief architect of one of the new biological paradigms of the twentieth century, stands out for what seems to me an explicit distaste for certain progressive social movements—including feminism that seeks to eliminate the "natural" differences between the sexes—and for directly linking sociobiology with his rejection of the social upheavals of the era.[10]

Sociobiologists have long sought to make all scholarship into branches of biology, reducing most human behavior to narrowly conceived Darwinian rules of evolution. Culture in this scenario remains a formal party to the human enterprise, but one created and governed by natural processes. Relying especially on neuroscience and evolutionary biology, human sociobiology asks, in Wilson's words, "What might the human instincts be? How do they fit together to compose human nature?" The take-home message is plain: "Human beings are guided by an instinct based on genes." As we will see, the idea of instinct is central to contemporary notions of male sexuality and aggression and to providing essentialist escapes out of gender confusion.[11]

When gender confusion brings doubt, the answer for Wilson has been to grasp the power of genes and heredity. Some allege that most of Wilson's science is solid and revelatory, and that his error is overzealous application in extending his claims. Whether or not this is true, Wilson's successors are partisans of what Richard Prum calls "bandwagon science." This history gives us reason to maintain a healthy bioskepticism when thinking about gender, sex, and sexuality.[12]

Like any important scientific treatise, Wilson's text was both a product of certain broader politics at play and a producer of them. The rise of sociobiology, as well as the storm of criticism that erupted in opposition to its tenets, and those of its successor, evolutionary psychology, was of a piece with its political times. In addition to Wilson's unnecessary comments about leftists of various eras, as evidence of the political views involved in his theory we might also consider this circumstantial evidence: the first generation of sociobiologists and its staunchest advocates were white southerners. The first generation of sociobiology's fiercest critics were northern Jewish leftists.[13]

We will return to Donald John Trump and the election of 2016 later. Here I want to consider the #MeToo movement and gender confusion, because although it was not simply an outcome of the election, #MeToo was easily among the most positive political developments to follow it. Yet as great an impact as the movement had, there were questions about gender that plagued politically progressive forces, contributing to flabbergasted exasperation and real gender confusion.

One question was: How could tens of millions of women vote for Trump, who on the campaign trail dared women to support him as a man's man, someone who was subject to no higher law than that shared by all naturally, sexually, and aggressively rapacious men? Some 63 million people chose Trump to lead despite the revelations of crude language and actions because they believed that if you let men off the leash that's just how they will behave, that it's in the basic makeup of all men to do so, even if some men are too timid to act on these impulses. For those who didn't agree with this analysis, well, they were deluding themselves with wishful thinking about men, and no doubt about many other things, too.

In trying to understand why so many women felt this way, it was easy to miss key elements of the particular historical period in which the election took place, especially the level of confusion, crisis, and anxiety with respect to gender that was being experienced broadly in the US population. Most election postmortems focused on economic and class concerns among the Trump electorate, but a major conservative backlash against women and gender progress was also underway, and it found shape as a central feature of Trumpian politics.

#MeToo was a reaction to Trump, but it was far more than that as well. If we recognize that the #MeToo movement happened simultaneously with millions of women voting for Trump, we can better view 2016 as a watershed moment of clash and confusion about boys and girls, men and women. And we can better appreciate why so many women did not recoil from the flagrant pussy-grabber, and in fact elected him to the presidency. At a moment of resurgent gender conservativism, when open hostility toward women is being promoted at the highest levels of society around the world, you might expect misogynist men to openly favor one of their own. But women? It is clear that underlying tenets about men and their sexuality and aggression provided these women with the logical explanation to elect this man: they all think about doing it, so get over it.

This moment has become not only a time of politically sanctioned assaults on women, but also a time of restless genders and shape-shifting men and women. Across the globe, "gender" and even "sex" are less stable terms than ever before. To better grasp the opportunities presented by this moment of gender uncertainty, agitation, and transformation, we need finer filters for our preconceptions about men and genetics, heredity, and bodily legacies. We need to be less surprised when men break an arbitrarily imposed mold.

GENDER CONFUSION ALWAYS

Let's return to the idea that males of all cultures and species seem to act in remarkably similar ways, and ask if this premise is true. It is possible to come up with strong universal (*but wrong*) definitions of men and masculinities. In all cultures, men need more sex than women do. We find the equivalents of mansplaining and manspreading throughout history. Human males are generally more irresponsible than females toward their offspring. Men more than women have been in control of politics, economics, and culture throughout history. Even though we find queens leading societies at various times, isn't it obvious to even the most casual observer that men have always run most institutions, in each and every corner of the globe? Such universal gender definitions must always be interrogated.

Here is the central wager of this book. If we can honestly conclude that men are so similar from one time to another and one place to another, then I am wrong, and some form of biological extremism is warranted. But if I am right, and such thinking is no more than persuasive folk wisdom, then we will need to reassess how we define masculinity and human maleness. I will make this bet because I have two powerful pieces of evidence on my side: variation and malleability.

Gender confusion is historical and cultural: many parts of the world have lived in steady-state confusion around gender and inhabited gender ambiguity with a lot less anxiety. The fact is that extremist claims on gender categories are mostly a matter of a provincial perspective. We in the United States are in some ways just catching up to the rest of the world in acknowledging how complex gender actually is or can be. That's why it's high time to get anthropological on the subject of men and masculinities by looking at three remarkable cases.

The *Muxe'* of the Isthmus of Tehuantepec, Oaxaca, Mexico

Flipping through the March 2007 issue of *Marie Claire* that one of my daughters left on the couch, I came across an article, "Meet Vidal Guerra & His Mother, Antonia: She's Turning Him into a Girl." The opening line read: "In Juchitán, Mexico, daughters are more valuable than sons. So mothers are encouraging their boys to become girls." In southern Mexico, the area known as the Isthmus of Tehuantepec is famous for how openly certain men, known as *muxe'*, cross-dress as women. They have sex with other like-minded men and also seduce younger men, sometimes for pay. Someone at the fashion magazine was evidently thrilled that a "traditional" indigenous society would host and promote such outré behavior in this mythical queer tropical paradise — How romantic! Erotic indigenes!

A common translation of *muxe'* is "transvestite gay man." But not all muxe' are gay. And some don't cross-dress. What the word means in daily life in the town of Juchitán defies this simple label. It refers to a creative form of social organization not found in many other parts of the world. Muxe' (pronounced *moo-SHAY*) are people who were born anatomically male, many of whom cross-dress, and, in the context of a fairly well-defined gendered division of labor, most of whom cross-work, too. Muxe' are not like other men. Some marry women and have children. More have relationships with men, and they sometimes continue to engage in these relationships even if they do marry women. The most common feature is that muxe' do women's work, from running the open-air markets to selling goods in the street to doing embroidery to making tortillas or jewelry.[14]

The intimate relationship between the muxe' and the women known as *Istmeñas* (the women of the Isthmus) is at the center of social life. Their role in the community together is legendary in the region, a mix of self-possessed and boisterous public personas. Tourist brochures often go overboard describing Juchitán as a matriarchy and a gay mecca, but the presence of Istmeñas and muxe' is striking and not found anywhere else in Mexico. Then there's the popular saying in the Isthmus that mothers favor muxe' sons, because muxe' will always be there to help their mothers.

Although the history of the muxe' is debated, many say this "third gender" long predates the conquest of the area by the Spanish in the early sixteenth century and the rigidly two-gender system the conquistadores brought with them. Though perpetually confusing to outsiders, the muxe' gender system provides local people of all kinds with a range of ways to embody gender in the world. At the same time, the mythology of the muxe' as it has been built up around the world has more to do with primordial sensationalism, imaginative sentimentality, and resourceful forms of being anatomical males but acting like females. At least for some muxe', some of the time.

The very impreciseness of what it means to be muxe' is itself part of what makes the identity dramatically different from two-gender norms in much of the world, where you are either male or female and there is general agreement about how that issue is settled. To be muxe' does not necessarily mean to be homosexual. But it can mean that, and often does. Moreover, the place of homosexuality in society as well as of men who cross-dress and cross-work is at the center of the social fabric in the Isthmus of Tehuantepec. "In Juchitán," wrote the poet Macario Matus, "homosexuality is regarded as a grace and a virtue that comes from nature." Although the outside world has overly romanticized Juchitán as a queer wonderland—homophobia there is still apparent, if more muted than in other parts of Mexico—the muxe' and the shifting relationship they have had for centuries within families and within the broader Isthmus society do indeed provide a clear example of long-term gender-bending ambiguity and indeterminacy.[15]

Sexual Initiation for Boys Among the Sambia of New Guinea

Some have called it "prolonged ritualized homosexuality"; others, child abuse. But no one has denied the historical reality of boy-to-man ritual practices among a people known as the Sambia who have long lived in the Eastern Highlands of Papua New Guinea. As anthropologist Gilbert Herdt, in particular, has documented, boys in the region are initiated as young as seven years old when they are taught, and forced, to perform fellatio on older boys.[16]

The rationale seems simple: in order to become men, they must have semen, and to get semen of their own they must first ingest the semen of older males, in this case older boys. At least until fairly recently, there were no Sambia men who had not gone through this initiation over a period of years. Otherwise they could not have become men. When they get older, the boys will in turn have younger boys who fellate them, until these boys become young men and old enough to marry women, at which point they will have sex exclusively with their wives.

This cultural pattern is so at odds with gender norms in the rest of the world that it is a very popular example taught in Introduction to Anthropology classes. If Sambia boys must fellate others, then get fellated, and then they stop any sexual contact with other males and devote their sexual energies to only women, what does this say about sexual orientation, identity, and trauma? About childhood and sexual cruelty? About childhood and erotic excitement? About male bodies, erections, semen, and male sexuality?

In one of his ethnographies on the Sambia, Herdt writes that "from such experiences is born a boy's sense of masculinity. Masculinity is thus a product of a regime of ritualized homosexuality leading into manhood." But, he points out, there is more than that involved, more than the symbolic transition from boyhood to manhood and the physical ingestion of semen. Indeed, Herdt insists that, "to be effective, male initiation must convert small, puny boys, attached to their mothers, into virile, aggressive warriors who are first erotically excited by boys and then by women." Herdt connects the underlying concept of gender and maturation among the Sambia to the erotic scripts they use in the process, which form severe demands on every participant at every stage.[17]

Respect it or despise it, consider it a set of ritual, sadistic, or erotic practices, the way in which Sambia males become men obliges us to reconsider what is natural and what is not about gender and sexuality among the males of any age or locale.

The *Hijras* of India

The nature of maleness and the fluidity of gender boundaries are also central to the lives of a group in India known as the *hijras*. The hijras are people born anatomically male who transition to a state in which they wear jewelry and women's clothing, remove facial hair, and grow their hair long. The most committed hijras renounce sexual desire. To achieve the highest status within their community, the renunciation must be sealed through castration.

That maleness is associated with sexuality and genitalia is not unusual in the world. That hijras seek to achieve spiritual purity by sacrificing their sex organs to a Hindu goddess, however, is. They take this path in order to gain the power to confer fertility to married couples and newborn babies, for example, and to participate in Muslim purification and burial rituals. Although some scholars have called hijras the "third gender" of India (as the muxe' of Mexico are sometimes labeled), others reject that notion altogether, arguing that hijras display a multiplicity of differences—sexual, religious, kinship, corporal—that do not fit neatly into a "third gender" category, much less a dualistic male-or-female framework. Though hijras show why pronouns matter, using she/her/hers over all others, even this concept is too limiting to encapsulate the multiple spaces they occupy in Indian society, some pious and some naughty.[18]

Hijras are known for two particular kinds of public displays: one is a stylized hand clapping, the other a forceful enactment of their ambiguous sexuality—lifting their saris to expose their genitals, or, better still, to show the space where their genitals used to hang. The flagrant exhibitionist act is meant to shock and confuse, to push passersby to question what it means to be a man, whether someone can be neither a man nor a woman nor even anything else quite so fixed and definable. Whether we view these acts of exposure as gender confusion being imposed on an innocent public or as a way of focusing attention on already existing, if rarely confronted, gender ambiguities, we would have to be ingenuous indeed not to see in these variations the kernels of a challenge to prevailing gender attitudes, relations, and practices on the themes of men and masculinities.

We should identify narrowness and naïveté as obstacles to understanding the possibilities of gender and the perils of gender conformity and of not appreciating the cultural phantasmagoria of what it means to be a man in the world. And we should also guard against the smugness of the idea that everyone else is stuck in narrow definitions about men and maleness, too unseeing to grasp that maleness is as much about possibility as about constraint.

Exploring the actual lives of men in places like Mexico, New Guinea, and India, we find so much variation in what it means to be a man, and in how masculinity is regarded, that it becomes far more difficult than we may have expected to offer neatly packaged characterizations of these concepts, and of what people who share male physiologies experience over the course of their lives. By acknowledging this variation, the long-standing and enduring diversity of ways that embody being a man, we can reassess maleness more fully—and more accurately.

GENDER CONFUSION AND DISTRESS

Gender confusion can lead to gender distress when old shibboleths about men and women no longer hold: it might seem as if, to quote Karl Marx, "all that is solid melts into air." For many, religion provides a mooring in times of confusion, which is why Marx noted that "religious distress is at the same time the expression of real distress and also the protest against real distress." In the same way that religion has long offered a solution to real distress, in our day science might seem a good way to think our way out of gender confusion and distress. In science we can find a way to explain and anchor whatever we are being forced to reconsider about men, maleness, and masculinity.

Marx, in discussing the comfort offered by religion, continued his consideration of real distress, writing, "Religion is the sigh of the oppressed creature, the heart of a heartless world, just as it is the spirit of spiritless conditions," and then concluded with this famous sentence, which is too often detached from the others preceding it: "It is the opium of the people." Usually this point is quoted to show how insulting Marx was toward religion. And he was quite critical of the role that organized religion, and religious ideas, had played in history. But he also had a deep grasp of why people find illumination and solace in religion; his writings showed an appreciation of the distress and despair of daily life that motivated people to seek insight and relief anywhere they could find them. Put in context, the "opium of the people" phrase shows an understanding of the lengths people go to in order to cope with social confusion and trauma. We should do no less in our quest to take account of extremist biological views on the meaning of men and masculinities: that is, while critiquing the real harm that such views can do, we should remember that they are ways of seeking insight and relief to cope with gender confusion and distress.[19]

Although, for understandings of maleness, conservatives and progressives do not represent two clear armies arrayed against each other, it is not difficult to discern general differences in how they regard certain issues, especially in terms of the relevance of our bodies (and animality) to the subject. The clearest line of demarcation concerns the extent to which we think gender is malleable, able to change, or, on the contrary, pretty well fixed by evolution and at birth.

A clear illustration of gender and flexibility is the fact that in 1900, in every national governmental body on earth, in nearly every large company, in just about every university, and in almost every other major social institution, men made up the entire leadership. At that time there were plenty of scientific rationales offered as to why this was the case. After all, if women were meant to lead, why couldn't we find any women leading anywhere at anything other than in a few monarchies here and there? It all seemed perfectly reasonable, rational, explainable, and permanent. The fact that men have continued to predominate in positions of influence in institutions around the world is of vital importance. That women increasingly exercise authority is even more significant, including as a fundamental refutation of naturalized excuses for women being excluded from power.

If the reason we still find far more men than women in positions of power is because it takes time and struggle to undo centuries of ingrained cultural patterns and prejudice, that's one thing. But if gender equality and getting women into power in essence represents an unwinnable fight against Mother Nature, then supporting women who seek to buck the gender fates is so much fanciful thinking.

Opposition to the notion of gender, gender relations, and gender identities being flexible persists with great acclaim, given the naysayers. In 2002, the best-selling author and psychologist Steven Pinker wrote, "By now many people are happy to say what was unsayable in polite

company a few years ago: that males and females do not have inter-
changeable minds." Along the same lines, and moving south from the
brain, an acquaintance once informed me, "What's all the gender confusion? If they'd just pull down their pants I could settle the mystery
about who's a man and who's a woman."[20]

Okay, I'll bite: What difference does it make if you are male or female? Are these male-female categories fixed? In what sense are these
categories important to our individual, social, and political lives? And
who gets to make these decisions? By insisting that men's and wom-
en's minds are really quite discrete, Pinker insinuated that fundamental
physiological gender differences are once again being well received by
scientists and the broader public, and that despite the changes that for-
merly occurred in people's thinking and attitudes, we should be happy
to be drawn back to the basics. Pinker believed that the latest findings
in cognitive science had proved once and for all that men are barely
removed from prehistoric animal urges and instincts, and among the
implications of this assertion was his vigorous defense of the idea that
rape by men is natural.[21]

Pinker is not confused about gender. His popularity stems partly
from the fact that he feeds off stale preconceptions about boy-girl differences and, using the imprimatur of science, feeds things back to a public
eager to hear confirmation of what they already suspected about men,
women, Mars, and Venus. Pinker is banking on the fact that his ideas
give scientific credibility to the prevailing outlook that human societies
have evolved according to natural laws.

Conservative thinking about men and their nature is capacious
enough to incorporate not only scientists like Pinker but also a range
of religious groups who do not suffer from any confusion about men
and masculinity. Far from representing some relics from the past, in the
United States key religious groups are imposing increasingly rigid gender demarcations in their canon. Some called it getting back to basics
when, for example, the Southern Baptists changed their rules in 2000 to
bring them more into sync with how God made men and women differ-

ently. Prior to 2000, there were no explicit restrictions on women holding the office of pastor. But that year, in the 18th Article of Baptist Faith
and Message, the elders ruled, "A wife is to submit herself graciously to
the servant leadership of her husband even as the church willingly sub-
mits to the headship of Christ." Biblical verses were invoked, including
1 Corinthians 14:34: "Let your women keep silence in the churches."[22]

The cause of these changes lay less with some new theological
revelation and more with the church's mandated response to an increasing unease and confusion about gender, control, and decision
making. The doctrinal changes reflected in good measure how the
church was—and is—coping with pervasive gender confusion and distress: with a resounding call to tighten up definitions and regulations
for living life in a neatly binary, hierarchical gender world.

The fact that these Bible verses have been around for some two
millennia, and presumably the church leadership had read them before, was never explained when the recent changes were made. Something in 2000 compelled these gentlemen to buttress the church's
recognition of gender differences and hierarchies, and that something
was a backlash against perceived challenges to the gender dimension
of God's grand design. In no way have the Southern Baptists shown any
compunction in answering the gender confusion of followers with anything other than an absolutist credo relegating women further under
the authority of their husbands and church elders.[23]

Neither Pinker and his like-minded scientists nor Southern Baptist
patriarchs and their like-minded brethren have taken a liking to the
renegotiation of gender categories. They have insisted instead that we
renew our commitment and belief that biology and/or God can better
extricate us from all such muddle and angst. Some atheists and non-
religious conservatives sound a lot like the religious right when they talk
about gender, substituting DNA for God as a way to explain the myster-
ies of life. They insist that deviation from a "traditional" understanding
of gender is ridiculous. These versions of biology (and the Bible) assert
you are male or female, and ambiguity is a delusion.

We could dismiss all this as the fringe views of marginal commentators, especially when we hear the even more lunatic warnings among certain of this ilk that transgender children are part of Satan's plan and that same-sex marriage will lead inevitably to bestiality. We need to take notice of these ideas because they have millions of believers; moreover, we may share some of the premises about stubborn underpinnings, such as begrudging appreciation that there is really something physically compulsory and universal about men's bad behavior.

Perhaps we just get lazy with our language, not fully realizing the implications of our metaphors. Unwitting assumptions about core differences between males and females are prevalent both in the inferences we make and in the way we conduct our daily lives. You may have heard (or thought), "Like it or not, I have to admit my boy and girl seem to be just so different by nature." Nonetheless, recent studies show that from birth parents treat newborn boys and girls differently—for example, in how we hold them, how much we hold them, how we manipulate their arms and legs, and how we talk with them.[24]

OUT OF CONFUSION

If the gender world appears simplistically binary, radical correction may be required for our cross-eyed disorder, to overcome our double vision. Gender confusion is not something to fear. We need to wrestle with it, not quixotically hope it will disappear. Welcoming new ways of thinking and talking about masculinity is possible and especially urgent in times of widespread uncertainty about what it means to be a man. We should be more skeptical of conventional narratives about men and masculinities.

There is nothing necessarily lazy about language that labels men and masculinity. Depending on what is meant, the term "toxic masculinity," for example, can be a useful way of talking about pernicious forms of acting like a man. But expressions that naturalize masculinity are problematic and often contribute to further confusing what men are and can be.

These phrases are often tongue-in-cheek, though never entirely so: "Be a man!" "Take it like a man!" "Grow a pair!" "Man up!" They convey a gap between the target of the injunction and some fetishized version of a man.

Yet there is more at play than phrases. The real problem is thinking that maleness is something instinctive, inherent, natural, essential, built in, and intrinsic to men. We reassess men and masculinities not mainly because men have been mistreated and maligned, or targeted unfairly. We do it because in times of gender confusion if the renegotiation of maleness and gender overall is premised on rooting maleness in extremist versions of the natural gender order of things, our mission is doomed from the beginning.

Continuing to act as if men's biology is their destiny is the problem. Renegotiating what it means to be men is the answer.

CHAPTER TWO

THE SCIENCE OF MALENESS

There are years that ask questions and years that answer.

Zora Neale Hurston

W E WERE SO INNOCENT IN 2002. THAT YEAR AN ADVERTISEMENT appeared in *Business Week.* The ad asked sympathetically, "Fatigued? Depressed mood? Low sex drive? Could be your testosterone is running on empty."

The makers of AndroGel wanted us to know there was a solution to our problems. Before, only a sliver of the population had been diagnosed with testosterone deficiency. By 2012, sales of the gel and other testosterone replacement therapy (TRT) medications aimed at boosting "Low T" had grown to $2 billion in the United States. By 2017 this figure was $5 billion, and it was expected to reach at least $6.5 billion in 2020. To put TRT sales in perspective, before its patent expired, worldwide sales of cholesterol-lowering Lipitor in 2010 amounted to around $5 billion. What accounts for this explosion of prescriptions is a stark illustration of the connections in the popular imagination between men's biology and men's well-being, desires, needs, and happiness. AndroGel didn't cause the Low T earthquake, but the company knew how to ride the resulting tsunami.[1]

In the late 1990s, Swedish and US pharmaceutical companies introduced the first TRT hormonal patch and gel, thereby leading the way with the express purpose of relieving men of their anxieties about growing older. Maybe it wasn't pushy women sapping men's virility after all, but a chemical imbalance. Men confused about their fatigue, diminished erections, and male-pattern hair loss had no further to look than their corner drugstore. Did endocrinologists and urologists working with AndroGel and their marketing teams manufacture a phony Low T crisis? Even if they did, they were simply the latest in a long line of biologists and medical practitioners to identify some part of the male body as the essence of maleness and take measures to address concerns about diminished manliness through medical intervention. Furthermore, what has been done with men and testosterone supplements since the late 1990s pales in comparison with efforts to adjust women's levels of estrogen to "solve" a multiplicity of diagnosed health issues.[2]

THE RISE OF LOW T

The science of maleness existed way before the discovery of hormones and testosterone, and newer branches of the science of maleness will continue to grow after hormones lose their cachet. But before we get to those, let's look more closely at the symptoms of Low T in men in the late twentieth century. As the AndroGel ad illustrated, the most commonly named signs were a lowered sex drive, less energy, more fatigue, and middling erections—at least as compared to what men in their twenties experienced. We can explain the sudden epidemic of Low T—and the instant availability of Low T medications—in one of two ways. Either Low T was a real and often overlooked problem that was finally brought into the spotlight, or the crisis was contrived and marketed as such.[3]

The fact is that the widespread epidemic of Low T diagnoses was related to a particular moment in the 2010s when issues surrounding men's health led to a spike in pharmaceutical remedies on the market. The issues underlying this imagined medical emergency had been festering for a long time. Testosterone in the 2010s has a privileged spot at the table where we discuss what makes men and women different. Don't they have very different levels of testosterone? It's an easy word to use: testosterone. It almost sounds like a sunscreen, or a chocolate bar. It's a shortcut for explaining both declining energy among older men and misconduct among younger men—or men of any age being crude. We reify our intuitions by giving behavior a chemical cause. An alarming number of contemporary discussions of masculinity spiral around the presumed properties of testosterone in one way or another.

The frenzy for TRTs developed by appealing to male vanity on late-night television and was legitimized through the creation of medical-sounding terms like "andropause." This and other additions to the lexicon were used to convince men they needed to remedy a disease they didn't even know they had. An advertisement for a product called Nugenix played on men having once been "A Fountain of Energy, Strength, and Vitality." But, "One day you wake up and realize you're just a shell of the man you used to be." It's not a man's fault—at least as long as he does something about his situation, once he realizes what his symptoms and options are. Nugenix boasted that it tapped into "nature's secret weapon," providing men with a "Free Testosterone Booster." Sly dogs, those ad-meisters. The commercial ended with the kicker, "And, guys, she'll like the difference, too!"[4]

And just like that, broad sectors of the male population were charmed into consuming this magical extract, including recreationally, and their sagging fortunes were rejuvenated. Meanwhile, the brand of "male hormone" was ever more indelibly impressed on the term testosterone, despite the fact that women have the hormone, too, though in far smaller percentages. The new thinking strengthened what John Hoberman called the "hormonal folklore of our culture," paving the way for testosterone to become a "charismatic drug" of choice.[5]

Testosterone didn't even exist before 1905, or, better put, the term didn't. It was used for the first time that year. Early in the twentieth century, testosterone came to mean masculinity, scientifically and popularly. British neuroscientist Joe Herbert, writing in 2015, noted that most testosterone in men comes from the testis; he concluded that therefore the "testis is the source of most of what we term masculinity." Herbert thus provided the physiological link between two periods of the science of maleness, one lasting more than two millennia and the other barely a hundred years old.[6]

Before there were so-called sex hormones, there were, of course, gonads, of both the male and female persuasions. For centuries in the West, until the twentieth century, scientists believed the gonads were the command centers for maleness and femaleness. Goat and wolf testes were among the aphrodisiacs of choice with the ancient Greeks and Romans. Much later, in the early twentieth century, men suffering from the effects of aging even tried getting the testicles of other animals transplanted into their own bodies, leading to what was known as "the monkey gland affair." The displacement of the science of testes and the uterus by sex hormones was marked by the founding of the scientific journal *Endocrinology* in 1917. Gonadal hormones, androgens and estrogens, were now "conceptualized as the chemical messengers of masculinity and femininity." By the time testosterone was first synthesized in 1935, the replacement of the anatomical model of sex with the chemical one was complete: masculinity and femininity could be better isolated and measured through a new metrics of strictly sexed bodies.[7]

Testosterone has more to tell us about the contemporary science of maleness, especially with respect to sexuality and violence, topics we will explore in their own right in Chapters 4 and 5. Here we will simply consider the studies by scientists seeking links between aggression and testosterone. The Stanford neuroscientist Robert Sapolsky acknowledges a possible relationship and asks what we should do if we detect a correlation. First, he suggests that we determine if there is a true correlation by testing three hypotheses:

1. Testosterone elevates aggression;
2. Aggression elevates testosterone secretion;
3. Or neither causes the other.[8]

If pressed, Sapolsky predicted, most nonspecialists would place their bets on #1, assuming that men with higher levels of testosterone are predisposed to be more aggressive. Or, to put it another way, most people think that if they know a man with especially aggressive tendencies, then the chances are that he also has a higher-than-average level of testosterone circulating in his bloodstream.

But if you thought that, you'd be wrong. According to current research, if aggression and testosterone are linked at all, then the correct answer is #2: most of the time aggressive behavior comes first, and it then raises the level of testosterone in one's body.

For most of us most of the time, however, it turns out that testosterone levels by themselves "predict nothing about who is going to be aggressive." And that fact holds true unless testosterone levels are extremely high or low. Unless they are lower than 20 percent of normal (think castration) or twice the normal amount (think gym rats on steroids), testosterone levels are all but irrelevant at telling you who's going to pick a fight. The data cannot support a strong common link between testosterone and aggression. The reason people treat testosterone as a miraculous potion is that we live in the age of abject worship of all biological explanations about a person's conduct. Facile invocations of what we think is scientific fact to explain complex human behavior are all too common.[9]

Perhaps the most fascinating recent work on testosterone is mostly ignored in the popular media: higher levels of testosterone can be correlated with higher levels of generosity. Because testosterone may intensify particular preexisting behavior, it turns out that not only aggression but also generosity might fit in the pantheon of typical guy conduct. Why only aggression has been noted and popularized is not so much a question for science as it is for social analysis. Is generosity not considered manly? And if it isn't, why not? And is this true for all men, or for some more than others?[10]

Yet not all scientists are convinced of testosterone's benign manifestations. And if testosterone does impact behavior, some consider this an overall positive influence. Take the following from Cambridge don Joe Herbert:

> There's a very simple reason why most financial traders are young(ish) men. The nature of trading incorporates all the features for which young males are biologically adapted. . . . The whole set-up seems to have been designed for young men. All the actions of testosterone are echoed by the qualities required of a successful trader. It does seem remarkable that the artificial world of financial trading should so suit the innate characteristics of young males.

I wonder if it has occurred to Herbert that working on Wall Street or London's Canary Wharf might induce changes in neurotransmitters and endocrine disrupters, and not simply that successful traders are preselected for their already existing aggressive physiologies. The fact is that testosterone rises in teenage boys but we see no leap in teenage boy aggression.[11]

All this testosterone-fueled aggressiveness can have a negative side, Herbert allows, as he draws out other direct implications of the hormone: "As well as the imprint of biological inheritance, we see the tendrils of testosterone all over war, gangs, and fanaticism." Because testosterone in men is thus seen as elemental, neurological synapses are called upon to rein men in: "And the human brain has had to devise multiple ways of regulating, channeling, and optimizing the powerful effects of testosterone on male behavior through laws, religion, and customs." Herbert's approach here is part of his larger reasoning: that testosterone may not be good, but it is found in nature, and thus must be controlled rather than ignored.[12]

Despite ample evidence casting doubt on testosterone's influence on male behavior in the gym, bedroom, boardroom, or battlefield, scientists remain tellingly interested in the subject. Beginning in the 1990s, the science of testosterone burgeoned into a Golden Age of research on the hormone, at least based on the evidence of the greatly increased number of scientific papers on every imaginable correlation between testosterone and aggression that were published in the three following decades. This research has examined whether testosterone can reliably be considered an all-powerful chemical responsible for male moods, impulses, desires, and behavior, especially in relation to aggression and sexuality, as shown in Table 1, compiled originally by Robert Sapolsky.

Number of Scholarly Articles on "Testosterone/Aggression," Based on Web of Science Database Search, 1920–2020

	TESTOSTERONE/AGGRESSION
1920–1930	0
1930–1940	0
1940–1950	0
1950–1960	2
1960–1970	3
1970–1980	24
1980–1990	53
1990–2000	401
2000–2010	757
2010–2020	1070

SOURCE: Robert M. Sapolsky, *Behave: The Biology of Humans at Our Best and Worst* (New York: Penguin, 2017), 605. (NOTE: 2010–2020 data are prorated from 2010–2015.) The table is reproduced here with Robert Sapolsky's kind permission.

As I see it, there are five possible reasons for the boom after 1990 in scientific literature on possible links between testosterone and aggression:

1. The growing number of articles on testosterone and aggression reflects more federal funding for research on testosterone.

2. The growing number of articles on testosterone and aggression reflects more funding by pharmaceutical companies for research on testosterone.
3. There is more popular interest in male biology and behavior, and the growing number of articles on testosterone and aggression is a response to that.
4. The growing number of articles on testosterone and aggression reflects more scientific discoveries.
5. Maybe it's all a sinister alt-right con job by a conspiracy nut.[13]

Putting aside #5, as tempting as that one might be, #1 and #2 are demonstrably true, and #3 is arguably correct. So that leaves us with #4.

But #4 is not borne out by facts. There have been no major new discoveries of a link between testosterone and aggression. The fact that we cannot point to any new scientific breakthroughs on testosterone and aggression gives the whole game away. The expanding science of testosterone, and the science of testosterone's connection to aggression, is all based less on new science and more on new social pressures to find a biological cause for male aggression. If a link could be proved scientifically it would settle the argument about why men are violent. As a sign in a sex shop in China in the 1990s read, "Get rid of ignorance; head toward science."[14]

Today we probably take for granted, at least in some countries, that if we use the word "testosterone" people will have some idea what we mean. Not the endocrinology of its interactions with the rest of the body, not any of what constitutes the actual science of the substance. But the allegory, the reference to something physiological that is really a reference to something symbolic for most of us. It means men, it means virility, it means male vitality, it means aggression. Yet how many of us would have a clue how to find testosterone under a microscope? Big T has taken on a fabled life of its own thanks not so much to the marketing wizards, or even to our gullibility, but most of all because enough of us wanted to believe in a scientifically substantiated substance that signifies and magnifies masculinity and can be administered with a swipe of transdermal gel in the male armpit. And for god's sake, keep it out of the reach of women and children.

By the time most scientists agreed that testosterone wasn't a singular, miraculous Manliness Factor after all, it barely mattered. The scientific hypothesis that a single male hormone could be responsible for so many of the things our culture thinks of as raw masculinity, thus proving they're all connected and biologically valid, was just too persuasive. Continued conflation of masculinity with the hormone testosterone, both by scientists and in popular opinion, is one example of the fraudulence of biobabble, when terms get tossed around to explain and excuse behavior as "natural" because it fits into our existing templates of what is expected.[15]

CATCHPHRASES "R" US

"Boys will be boys," right? It's among the most common of phrases, a tired one-liner tossed into many a conversation as an offhand barb. It's used by men and women, by old and not-so-old, in every English-speaking region of the world. A half-joke, to be sure—it's rarely meant as pure and precise truth. But it is also usually not expressed as an entirely frivolous wisecrack. There's always an aspect of something thought to be real, something underlying people who are male of any age, something bordering on the irrepressible. Despite whatever parents might think is automatically different about their sons and daughters, however, it is unlikely to be hormonal, since throughout childhood—after infancy and before puberty—testosterone levels are similar in boys and girls. Yet "Boys will be boys" is a saying that is declared in an implicit appeal to mutual understanding and shared experience. What can you do, boys will be boys? No way around it, boys will be boys. Well, that explains it, because boys will be boys, won't they, after all? Isn't that just typical of boys being boys?

And the corollary: girls better watch out.

If biologists can explain major parts of our lives—from sexual behavior to militarism, from falling in love to sugar cravings, from cut-
throat marketing to anger management, then even if we do not like the
way nature has evolved, dammit, we have to respect it.

Genitalia have been at the center of scientific theories of sex differences since time immemorial. As we have seen, for much of the twentieth century, sex hormones ruled the science of sex difference. Most
recently, sex differences have been focused on genetics and the human
genome. With the sexing of genetics, writes historian of science Sarah
Richardson, "the tendency to see the sex binary as writ molecular in
the X and Y chromosomes is most evident in the gendering of the X as
female and the Y as male." It is perhaps only a matter of time before the
new science of proteomics (the large-scale study of proteins in a cell)
discovers the key to maleness and determines that masculinity lies in
one or another protein feature.[16]

Research on the Y chromosome began in the 1950s, and since that
time the Y has come to represent the essence of manhood in scientific
studies. As always, there has been a push-pull influence on the science
of maleness, with preexisting beliefs about gender and sex inspiring
the research, and the research confirming the original bias. Indeed,
early on, in the 1960s, the focus of 82 percent of studies on the Y chromosome was on an alleged link between aggression and men who had
two Y chromosomes, not one, known as XYY men. Genetics research
at that time had come to the firm conclusion that if a man had too
much Y, he was likely to be more violent. The science behind this
hypothesis held sway for nearly two decades. But then, with further
research, the theory was suddenly and thoroughly disproved. By 1980,
XYY men had disappeared from the scientific literature. They were
no longer the poster boys for biological explanations linking violence
and men.

Since the completion in 2003 of the Human Genome Project, the
biology of sex has centered on genetics and chromosomes. Despite the
fact that the Y chromosome is by no means the only place to find genes

relevant to maleness, in both scientific and popular literature the association of the Y chromosome as the new base camp of maleness persists.
In a case of disrupting the neat two-dimensional model of sexual differentiation, for example, estrogen, the so-called female hormone, is also
involved in the development of male brains. As Sarah Richardson put
it, "each time a new research program emerges, the claim is made that
at last the difference between the sexes can be located, measured, and
quantified, and that the differences between the sexes are greater than
ever previously imagined."[17]

The seeming objectivity of the laboratory lends respectability to the
science of maleness. It is hard to argue with biological facts, and if they
verify preexisting ideas about men and masculinity, so much the better.
Scientists have a name for finding what you are looking for whether it is
there or not: confirmation bias. We know boys will be boys, and when
science tells us that boys will be boys because of biology, then boys will
be boys becomes scientifically certifiable.

Each new scientific theory about maleness echoes contemporary
cultural mores about men and masculinity and enhances the science
of maleness. Our assumptions about universal qualities and behaviors
of men (just like other stereotypes) are very often particular to a time
and place. What is expected of boys and girls, men and women, varies
greatly by geography and historical period, including when it comes to
men's sexuality and aggression. Our cultural environments affect our
thinking, no matter who we are or what we do. Scientists are no more
immune to that cultural environment than the rest of us, and they, too,
can reinforce preexisting, mistaken ideas about life.

Yet much of the power of the science of maleness is that each of its
theories seems to unravel prior confusion and mystery about why men
do what they do. Some of the appeal of the science of maleness relies
on what novelist Joyce Carol Oates called "nature mysticism," which
she defined as "Nature adoration; Nature-as-(moral)-instruction-for-
mankind." If only we could understand what nature *wants* from men,
we could then live better as men and with men, more fully in tune with

natural man. Or at least we could better understand how we *should* live as and with men.[18]

There are plenty of grounds for optimism that we are witnessing a rapprochement between studies of biology and culture in the early twenty-first century. Emerging fields like epigenetics and neuroscience hold great promise that we can find new language to describe human experience in a more holistic fashion, whether we call the fusion bio-sociality, sociogenomics, cultural epigenetics, or biocultural synthesis, and whether we draw attention to the social in biology or to the bioso-cial turn. This is potentially big news. Too often throughout the twen-tieth century, the biological sciences and social sciences were talking past each other as they worked mostly in autonomous regions of inquiry. This hurt the science of maleness as well as the science of human rela-tionships. Even in anthropology, with its claim to bridge the biological and social through specialists in both fields housed in the same depart-ments, in reality we have at best been good at parallel play.

Recent work on both sides of the anthropological aisle has spurred renewed efforts to link the cultural and biological. Mexican social theo-rist and anthropologist Roger Bartra, for example, argues that the mallea-bility of cultural and social networks facilitates a "prosthetic" connection to the brain and consciousness. But, he writes, "we cannot accept the idea that there is a moral module in the central nervous system, capable of determining the ethical considerations of individuals."[19]

If extreme male sexual and violent conduct is prompted by malfunc-tioning brain chemicals or limbic encephalitis or misfiring synapses, then this conduct cannot be prevented or altered by legal statute or so-cial opprobrium. It's no use fighting factors beyond our control: if men are aggressively sexual and violent by nature, and that nature is fixed, we have little to gain by trying to change them, or by expecting them to be capable of change. For problems that are deemed intractable and irresolvable, one can only hope to keep them under control—if men are obligatorily aggressive, we need to simply corral them, if indeed they can be contained and restrained.

In the United States and other countries there is a long history of science advancing theories about the abilities or lack of abilities among particular sectors of the population. In the early twentieth century, "scientific racism" was a powerful framework in academia and the popular press—both nearly all white—and racial differences were casually and routinely attributed to intrinsic physical and immutable traits that had the imprimatur of scientific research. As historian Richard Hofstadter wrote of scientists in the twentieth-century who stretched the relevance of biology beyond its reasonable limits, "so authoritative did their biological data seem" that the lay public could easily be cowed by their lack of expertise.[20]

In the twenty-first century, few scientists give public credence to scientific theories of racial superiority and inferiority. The same cannot be said of the acceptability of the theories about men and women, and for rationalizations supposedly proven by research for their differential achievements. The support for false claims among scientists can in turn impact what the broader public thinks. Researchers Barbara Duden and Silja Samerski call it "the effect of laboratory language in everyday life." It is getting worse, and we should know why.[21]

We should explore and account for the popular enthusiasm for the putative scientific beliefs that lead so many people to the conviction that men as a group have minimal control over their sexual and violent "natures" and that they must be managed and restrained, usually by societal restrictions or by the women in their lives. A folk biological narrative can be compelling when trying to understand the gendered undercurrents in the biological explanations about human behavior that are pervasive in various societies today.

Nonetheless, the biology of maleness may be more remarked upon than understood. Why and how our thoughts and opinions can seek validation in words like "anatomy," "genes," and "gonads," why and how they hold sway in the popular imagination in otherwise very different kinds of societies, and why and how, especially at this particular historical moment, these ideas are in the air we breathe, could be primarily the outcome of new scientific discoveries in the past few decades. Or not. What social factors impinge on our science and scientific explanations of human relationships, especially with respect to the inner natures of men and boys?

If the aptitudes and interests of men and women are largely distinct, fixed, permanent, and rooted in biology, then any semblance of social equality between the sexes is a pipe dream. Yet let's use caution before accepting this conclusion too readily. As biologist Anne Fausto-Sterling writes, "there are very few absolute sex differences and . . . without complete social equality we cannot know for sure what they are." If we have accomplished nothing else through the science of maleness in the past hundred years, we have learned that even apparently absolute physical disparities between men and women—for example, in hormone levels, brain wiring, athletic abilities—are in good measure the consequences of social relationships, restrictions, and opportunities. Every time a social barrier to gender equality has been removed, lo and behold, women and men look more similar to each other than before in meaningful ways.[22]

MURDERERS ARE MEN

In later chapters I will discuss beliefs about the origins, explanations, and implications of male violence more fully. Here I want to briefly look at relevant recent work on the science of male violence. By recognizing that most murderers are men, for example, we must know that the stakes are far higher here than in our considerations of erectile dysfunction and questions about why boys play with trucks.

Worldwide, about nine men commit murder for every one woman who does. Can we glean any indication about an underlying physical condition of maleness that leads to violence? Are men necessarily nine times more violent than women? One leading authority on the biology of violence, Adrian Raine, thinks so, concluding, simply, "Men are murderers." Yet as Raewyn Connell, a leading scholar of men and masculinities, has written, "almost all soldiers are men, but most men are not soldiers. Though most killers are men, most men never kill or even commit assault. Though an appalling number of men do rape, most men do not. . . . There are many non-violent men in the world. This, too, needs explanation."[23]

It would certainly seem at times that Raine is right. In an era of frequent, highly publicized mass shootings, we have learned that the perpetrators are nearly always male. What is it, then, about men and their violent appetites?

Murder may appear to be rooted in universal male traits, but Connell also has a point: most men are not murderers, and we need to account for this. If we don't—if we pin murder, rape, and other forms of violence on male biology—we could end up treating men as victims of their own bodies and doing nothing about it.

Male biology is often the alleged accessory to the crime in cases of interpersonal violence. But what about violence foisted on the world by politicians and generals? In that case, it's often considered a "good and necessary violence" linked to intelligent strategy, and sometimes, genius. We view global movers, shakers, and policy makers as manifesting their analytical functions in warfare in the name of freedom, democracy, or national security. It is socially sanctioned.

In the United States, we also need to explain the fact that in 1991, the murder rate was 20.8 per 100,000 people, while in 2008 it was 11.3 per 100,000. (The percentage of male murderers remained the same.) Furthermore, we need to explain the following findings from the United Nations Office on Drugs and Crime in 2014: "Intentional homicide caused the deaths of almost half a million people (437,000) across the world in 2012. More than a third of those (36 percent) occurred in the Americas, 31 percent in Africa and 28 percent in Asia, while Europe (5 percent) and Oceania (0.3 percent) accounted for the lowest shares of homicide at the regional level." Beyond differences in population size, surely we are past arguing for the notion that human males in Samoa and São Paulo are biologically distinct, yet that is just where an essentialist argument on men and violence can lead.[24]

The same 2014 UN report notes that in Haiti, the homicide rate doubled over a period of five years, going from 5.1 to 10.2 per 100,000 between 2007 and 2012. Could it be that the devastating 2010 Haiti earthquake and ensuing social turmoil, such as increased gang violence, caused Haitian men's physiologies to transform to such an extent? We will look in subsequent chapters at the issue of the behavioral factors involved in changing biologies, but no environmental factors have ever been shown to dramatically change people's bodies in a way that would explain the doubling of homicides in Haiti in five years.[25]

It gets worse. Not only are key scientific findings used retroactively to explain why men have murdered or raped; they are also used prospectively to purportedly show why some men are more likely to murder than others based on physical attributes. The same University of Pennsylvania scholar who pointed out that nine out of every ten murderers are men is also a big advocate of measuring fingers to see which men are likely to be most aggressive. Specifically, Adrian Raine argues, we need to measure the difference between a man's index finger and his ring finger (palm up), because by doing so we can predict manliness among men: the longer the ring finger as compared to the index finger, the more "male-like" the man. A joke? Hardly. The "2D:4D" (for second digit to fourth digit) ratio is widely promoted among scientists, including sharp critics of biological determinism.

Professor Raine continues: "What do we know about people with a more male-like, longer ring finger? For one thing they tend to dominate, show physical advantages, have male-like characteristics, and have personalities linked to aggression. . . . Another correlate of the long ring finger is sensation-seeking and impulsivity." Moreover, "men with a longer ring finger tend to have higher attractiveness ratings," whereas "gay men's ring-finger lengths are often in between those of heterosexual men and heterosexual women." Needless to say, what constitutes "gay" is never defined. Would that we all fit so neatly into these simplistic categories.[26]

For the denouement, we move on from simple manifestations of masculinity, interpersonal aggression, and gayness to geopolitics. "If you were the leader of a country," Raine proposes, "and in conflict with your neighbor over diamond mines [cue, image of African dictators] that had just been discovered in disputed territory, how would you react? Suppose you can either negotiate or go to war. Your choice is not entirely as free as you may think. It's partly determined by your relative ring-finger length." Drawing out explanations about male sexuality and violence from the basket of anatomical features is hardly a sign of ignorance versus knowledge. Some very learned people treat our bodies as fonts to decipher our social arrangements and in the process, intentionally or not, confound our very understanding not so much of bodies as of societies themselves.[27]

From men as murderers to men as sexual assailants, these ideas are inescapable. Consider a news item from November 29, 2016: in a survey by the Canadian government's statistical agency, more than 25 percent of women in the Canadian military reported that they had been sexually assaulted during their careers. But only 23 percent of those who said they had been assaulted reported the assault to their military supervisors. It is not hard to see why. To understand problems like sexual harassment, according to the former chief of the Canadian defense staff, General Tom Lawson, we need to recognize that "it's basically because we're [that is, men are] biologically wired in a certain way and there will be those who believe it is a reasonable thing to press themselves and their desires on others. It's not the way it should be." Lawson later apologized, and indicated men should not assault women. Still, one wonders if he did not believe what he had said about men being physically compelled to assault women, and regretted saying it, or was just disappointed by the public's inability to concede what (for him) was a clear-cut matter of biological fact.[28]

THE SCIENCE OF MALE ANIMALS

The scientific language of maleness extends the appeal of biological truthiness from androgens to Y chromosomes to 2D:4D finger measurements. But nowhere do we find the lexicon of maleness more in evidence than when the gents of various species are compared with each other.

Men are called pigs, and also wolves, snakes, and dogs. Seldom are they compared to gazelles or ospreys or dolphins. It's hard to miss the message: not all animals are people, but all people are animals. And, so what? Because humans share 98 percent of their DNA with chimpanzees— or so begins the circular argument based on the assumption that our DNA governs what we think, say, and do: if male chimps are aggressive a lot of the time, and if chimp groups are run by alpha males, why, then, there must be a genetic clue as to why humans go to war and why men predominate in positions of power in every society on earth. It's in the DNA we share with the chimps.[29]

Like the purveyors of social tolerance, the biologists of behavior might claim the neutral high ground as they adjudicate what is biological, and therefore supposedly beyond culture, and as they position their cultural critique as aimed primarily at the religionists. We need to ask ourselves if the substitution of DNA for God is a step forward or the replacement of one blanket prescription for another. Undoubtedly, it might seem more fashionable to summon up scientific terms when you're gossiping with friends about that sexually ambiguous neighbor of yours.

But what does it mean to talk about that friend of yours, the one with the appendage that seems to have a mind of its own? And why do men have attachments that have minds of their own, but women do not in any analogous way? And what does all this say about men as a group being more governable by their natures—you could even say, by their animal natures? Men are animals. Again, so what?

One area where disputes about universal and unique traits take place concerns animals. For various reasons, many ethologists who study the science of animal behavior like to use words about human behavior to describe the activities of nonhuman animals. They're catchy. And they make memorable parallels, deserved or not, between humans and nonhuman animals, and, more fundamentally, between the supposed evolutionary origins of male and female sexual behavior across species.

To put a check on such metaphors, I think we need more bioskepticism, more willingness to counter the quasi-religious belief that biological makeup is the key to the universe of animals of all stripes, the cryptic code, the "Open Sesame!" we can and should use to understand all human and nonhuman male animal behavior. Unlike its cousin, bioworship, bioskepticism requires a finely specialized knowledge of things. A convert's trusting disposition will not suffice. Bioskepticism is not against science any more than it is against biology. Nor does it insist that you seditiously ignore expert wisdom. It does entail a certain denial of "the will of nature," and it does challenge the idea that every important matter across the kingdom—including sexuality and mating, competition and authority, violence and aggression, nurturing and fostering—can be explained better by biology than by anything else.

The science of maleness throughout the twentieth century and into the twenty-first has proved time and again that social values and expectations exert undue influence on our findings, whether they be unwarranted comparisons of human males to males of other species or specious links between chemical cocktails in male bodies and aggression. At this point, every time we hear someone expound on male behavior by appeal to biological reasoning, maybe it wouldn't hurt if our initial response was suspicion instead of credulity.

Provocative tags for animal behavior may be a way for students of animal behavior to remember certain responses to stimuli they cannot control, much less evaluate, but they can also serve to legitimize the understanding that these behaviors are hardwired. It all starts in childhood, with pets, stuffed animals, and animal shows on TV. You might think none of these is exactly scientific. Nonetheless, they all provide evidence-based animal accounts. And one especially scientific-seeming way of talking about men is to find similarities between males of various species.

CHAPTER THREE

MONKEY SEE, HUMAN DO

*I'll say it again: imitating human beings was not
something which pleased me. I imitated them because
I was looking for a way out, for no other reason.*

FRANZ KAFKA, "A Report to an Academy,"
concerning the narrator's previous life as an ape

SIGMUND HAD A MONKEY. THAT'S HOW MY MOTHER ALWAYS BEGINS the story. The Sigmund in question was my great-great-grandfather Sigmund Oppenheimer, and as a boy I tried to invoke this precedent to convince my mother to let me get a chimpanzee. Having a primate was a birthright.

Sadly, the denouement of the family monkey saga did not help my case. The creature (whose name has been lost in the family memory) would follow Sigmund around the house doing what monkeys do, aping his human. This included sitting on my great-great-grandfather's shoulder as the old man shaved. My mother did not shield me from the tragic conclusion to this family tale. As you may have already guessed, one day when Sigmund was at work the monkey found the razor and, no doubt trying to emulate his human male, shaved for the first and last time.

It is not a mistake to think about men in relation to the males of other animal species. Such cross-species comparisons provide an especially accessible lens through which to understand what might be expected from males of all kinds. That we're all animals and that we all come from common ancestors, way back when, is a bedrock understanding of life on earth. The raw intelligence of an elephant should awe us, but not surprise us, and when we underestimate the human-like qualities of other animals we do them a tremendous disservice. If the similarities were tested rigorously, we might find productive reference points to help in dissecting gendered issues among humans, including sex and violence. But caution is also warranted, because the significance of animals in our lives, and the ratification by science of what we believe is special about male animals, can lead us all too easily to exaggerate the extent to which men do things because they are male, almost as if they can't help themselves.

We give human names to the nonhuman animals we keep closest, the ones who are practically part of the family. It is a way of marking the intimacy of our encounters. I wish I could give you the name of Sigmund's monkey. We've put the family lineage maven on the case, but so far nothing has turned up from Ellis Island registries or Amazonian bills of lading.

Other than watching them at zoos, the closest I've come to communing with monkeys has been to live vicariously through primatologist colleagues, who study animals in forests, savannahs, and jungles, and are kind enough to return with their chronicles from the wild. When the primatologists recount their scientific parables, we learn of bizarro habits and routines along with the theories linking them to other species, best of all the human varieties. One hazard we need to avoid when it comes to comparisons with animals is cherry-picking from the animal smorgasbord when one or another similarity helps us make some broader point about human relationships. It is one thing to make animal comparisons to prove the validity of evolution. It is another to use them to shed light on human behavior today, as a mirror onto our own ways of mating, parenting, provisioning, fighting, and reconciling. Here we need special caution, because while there are abundant similarities, and greater knowledge of nonhuman animals does enhance our appreciation for their own complexities, we need to avoid falling into simplistic models for human behavior, including male sexuality and aggression.

The fact is that animal behavior is too multifaceted and varied to use as a trouble-free mirror on human activities. The greatest pitfall of overly inflating the coincidence of interests and activities of humans and other animals is that we can mistakenly ignore the context-specific environments in which all these pursuits take place. It is one thing to gain new awareness of the manifold splendors of nonhuman animals. It is another to reduce humans to one end of a one-dimensional animal continuum in the name of natural selection.

LEARNING FROM PETS AND THE DISCOVERY CHANNEL

A lot of what we learn as children about male behavior we learn through animals. Male dogs lift their legs to mark territory; tomcats can get aggressive when encountering one another. One of the results of urbanization throughout the world has been that people rarely have contact with nonhuman animals except as pets. Even if you didn't grow up with pets—and chances are decent you did, because in 2018, Americans had 90 million dogs and 86 million cats—from childhood you read books featuring animals talking to each other and doing funny things, and watched television programs that featured animals, especially talking cartoons and nature programs that described the animals' fears, hopes, and motivations. You had names and personalities for your stuffed animals. As an adult, you adopt a pet that feels like a family member, or marvel over the human-like antics of horses and goats.

Yet projection is a two-way street. Not only is our understanding of human male behavior filtered through our experience with nonhuman animals, but our study of nonhuman biology is deeply affected by our understanding of human males and females. And, not surprisingly, in virtually all serious accounts of male and female animal behavior, Charles Darwin is employed as a scientific talisman to wave over evolutionary tales, tall and other, about nature, nurture, and culture.

There are parallels with how we talk about people: sometimes we lump all humanity together, emphasizing commonalities despite superficial differences in appearance. In the same way, sometimes there is a point in lumping all animals together to trace their common evolutionary origins. The accent here is on shared phylogenetic origins, endocrinology, and ethology, our common humanity, animality, and shared life on earth.

But lumping has its problems. Sometimes generalizing about humans conceals meaningful differences, specifically inequalities. People can be different in virtue of the different ways they suffer, because of whom they love, or whether they pray five times a day or not at all. Erasing these complexities creates a false equivalence and can inadvertently reveal a lot about what different cultures do and do not value. So, too, with simplistic comparisons between humans and other animals.[1]

Our fascination with nonhuman animals, *zoophilia*, comes in boundless forms. Sometimes even a casual observation belies underlying cognitive schema about men's animality. My friend Roberto in Mexico City gave me a tutorial on human-animal associations one day as he repaired radiators with his acetylene torch. With a fun-loving smirk, he tested my manly expertise when it came to wooing women.

"What does a woman need to feel complete, Mateo?" I responded by asking Roberto to educate me. "First, a cat in the kitchen," Roberto said, adding, in case I couldn't follow the allusion, "That's someone who can help her with the cleaning and food." He continued, "Second, a Jaguar at the door. That means a good car. Third, a tiger in bed. And fourth, an ox who supports her!" Only a true renaissance man, an all-around animal man, could satisfy a woman's every need.[2]

But the zoophile's poster boys are surely male primates, who are often presented to the public as displaying a range of unfortunate truths about mammalian maleness, siring, fathering, neediness, bossiness, and malevolence, along with a healthy dose of petulance. Bonus points when claims about silverbacks can be made apropos of their human male counterparts. Bruce Springsteen speaks for many of us when he sings, "Part man, part monkey, baby that's me."[3]

We have looked already at the science of maleness. Now we delve further into exaggerated claims of correspondence among males throughout the animal kingdom. The goal is not so much to avoid normative ways of thinking about male humans as to question what we take to be the norms for masculinity: men are far more flexible than an overdetermined biology of man allows. When we embellish the commonalities shared by males across species, we make ourselves more susceptible to a cross-eyed perception that the gender binary is as homogeneous for humans as it may be for other animals.

Children can learn about male and female from pets, television, and sometimes even stuffed animals. If they live in a city where most youths make it through high school, chances are they will pick up some basics of genetics and endocrinology along the way, including what their textbooks teach them about the importance of Y chromosomes, androgens, and estrogens. But for many, television nature programs are the most comprehensive source of information about animals and the science of maleness they will encounter. These shows are ubiquitous and available around the world. Television programs about nature are foundational for contemporary knowledge about boys and girls, birds and bees.

I know a retired factory worker in Shanghai whom everyone calls Teacher Li. When I asked him what he thought was different about men and women, he replied, nonchalantly, "hormones." When I asked what he meant by this, Teacher Li replied, "Men's hormones go up when they see pretty women." When I asked Teacher Li where he came up with this idea, he told me, "Television, of course." He was an avid fan of the nature shows that had become available in post-reform China.

As of 2017, the Discovery Channel claimed to reach over 400 million households in more than 170 countries, surpassing its media stepsister Animal Planet's 90 million households. In recent decades, these shows have grown tremendously in popularity. As measured by reach, engagement, revenue, and the all-important "mind share," Discovery Channel and Animal Planet by 2017 were winning among numerous demographic sectors and in various time slots for leisure viewing around the globe. Arguably the core lessons of these shows and the zany animal antics they present is, "Hey, they're just like us!" Much of the world learns scientific and pseudoscientific information about animals and maleness from these channels.[4]

Nature programs tell us that piggish lotharios are common throughout the animal kingdom. Males of avian and mammalian species have some unvarying need to control their habitats, so maybe this is why societies look to men as the primary providers of hearth and home. It doesn't take a genius to see something human in the way male goats, tigers, and sea lions fight for territory, and how females choose the winners of these contests as their sexual mates. These shows often find the same patterns of male behavior across the animal kingdom, and for many viewers there is some comfort to be found in that. Why are we so susceptible to suggestions that our own exploits, delusions, and desires are similar to what we've learned about mama bears and seahorses? Why does the notion of a sexually choosy male seem oxymoronic?

If people feel distress or confusion about gender relationships—for example, about men's wolfish ways—this is real anxiety, and it makes sense that we might look for answers in television. If men are animals, and problems between men and women evolve from natural causes almost beyond our ability to restrain, then our confusion and stress about what it means to be male can be made more palatable.

ANIMALS ARE GOOD TO THINK WITH

Let's readily acknowledge that animals are good to think about and with, and how often we do this as part of daily life. Animals are also good to swear with. Comparing someone to a nonhuman animal, as

British scholar Edmund Leach remarked years ago, comes behind only sex, excretion, and blasphemy when you're hurling invectives. Many of us sling around nasty animal analogies about males with great relish, often with a patina of naturalist rhetoric. In Spanish alone, men who are schmucks are called goats, lazy men are dogs, stupid men are donkeys, nasty men are pigs, and thieves are rats; a woman can be called a beast, a cow, and a foxy slut, and anti-revolution Cubans in Miami have been called worms. In China, you can call a male prostitute a duck and a female prostitute a chicken; ugly women are dinosaurs, ugly men are frogs; no one wants to be a turtle egg, and everyone expects children to be little monkeys. At the most extreme, biology and animality are held to practically dictate male behavior.[5]

Going back to Aristotle's *scala naturae*, or "ladder of being," defining the relationships between earth's living creatures has challenged philosophers and recreational thinkers alike. René Descartes held that animals resemble nothing so much as ignorant machines. He never saw an android, but he did talk about the animal machine, calling animals natural *automata*. Two centuries later, Charles Darwin declared that all species share progenitors, and that we humans are unambiguously animals. The differences, he held, are matters of degree.[6]

To philosophers and poets animals often represent nature in its purest state. This tendency often serves to highlight our fear that humans are nature's apotheosis, its biggest, cruelest failure. But the tenor of scientists is usually different. Animal studies and popular articles highlight apes that use sign language, dolphins that develop complex social strategies, and octopuses that manipulate tools to hide and defend themselves. They emphasize the animal in the human, and the humanity in the animal. For many researchers, a core issue has been whether "with rapid changes to human cultures in the last ten thousand years that far out-paced our ability to adapt physically . . . humans remained 'suited biologically' to the modern world." For them the study of other animals makes it clear that our human cultures can never escape our common animal natures.[7]

Anthropomorphism—giving nonhuman animals, ghosts, or gods human characteristics—is central to our understanding of the history and unity of the animal kingdom, humans included. Only creationists seriously question the validity of cross-species commonalities. Problems with such juxtaposing, wisely employed, might appear at first blush to lead us into nothing more knotty than whimsical thinking. The appeal to hyperrealism, biologies, compulsions, and ever more ineluctable organic arguments about what constitutes bedrock maleness across the animal kingdom gives rise to a paradise of metaphoric possibilities, "Men are pigs!" being only too obvious.

As children quickly learn in comparing themselves to animals, we all eat, breathe, poop, make babies, sleep, and a whole lot more. Nonhuman animals are in some ways just like us humans. From aardvarks to zebus, from the most domesticated to the wildest animals, there are an awful lot of similarities in how we move about in the world. The issue is not so much how important these commonalities might be, but which ones are important, why we find them important, and how they can lead our understanding of maleness astray.

Many of us believe we have a good idea of what a pet thinks and feels, for example—we delight in our pets' happiness and maybe feel a little guilty if they seem sad when we leave. We empathize with them, just as we're sure they empathize with us when we're sad. We can explain why we are fond of a particular species.

When Claude Lévi-Strauss said that "animals are good to think with," he was examining "totemism," an Ojibwa term signifying a kinship between particular groups of humans and special animals or plants that serve as their symbol, or totem. Central to the concept of totemism is an appreciation that nonhuman animals, too, have minds, and thus humans and totems can be linked through thought, although, as Emile Durkheim long ago wrote, totems really say more about human relations with each other. It was no small matter to associate the minds of human and nonhuman animals so directly, but Lévi-Strauss's purpose was different. He was not so much crossing species boundaries as he was out to prove a point about the minds of humans: that they are all the same. Nonhuman animals were good to think with, in part because they could help us recognize this fact about humans.[8]

The philosopher Thomas Nagel famously asked, "What Is It Like to Be a Bat?" The short answer was, who knows? Because humans surely cannot. Hang upside down in gravity boots like a bat, and you're a human swinging upside down with clamps around your ankles. Tap into your undeveloped potential for echolocation, as some blind people report they are able to do in order to sidestep obstacles, and you've managed to avoid a tumble. We don't pretend that because we humans and giraffes can walk that we know what it means to be a giraffe. Nagel's point is not that bat-ness doesn't exist, but that we cannot know what it is like to be a bat simply by looking at its behavior or studying its physiology.[9]

Imitation and imagination are central to the relationship between animals and humans, and not just for Disney. And what's wrong with a little animal whimsy? Who gets to say if parallels are reasonable and appropriate? In the recent theater of animality, we see wrangling over animal boundaries with special poignancy, as other creatures are woven into performances to great effect for vicarious and subversive ends. All manner of bestiality is conjured up to shock us into thinking better about males, sexuality, and what comes spontaneously. When we take away the clothing, are males really so different?

Ordinarily we might think that evolutionary psychology and theater have little in common. But when it comes to animals, especially of the male variety, playwrights can exploit the same kind of common assumptions and prejudices about male animals—for example, that the males of all species will screw just about anything they can get their hands on, and do so full of self-righteous justifications for their actions.

Consider for a moment how Edward Albee's *The Goat, or Who is Silvia?* projects human qualities onto an animal, the Silvia in question. Or does Albee have a human assume animal qualities? The plot rests on scandalizing social values guiding human-animal interactions, in what some call a theater of species, or a promotion of interspecies awareness. *The Goat* asks us to pity Martin and fear for him, a husband and father who with frenzied abandon is fornicating with Silvia, the ruminant in question. Martin insists he is helpless before the goat's bestial charms, finding himself especially captivated after he gets a chance to stare into Silvia's eyes: "She was looking at me with those eyes of hers and . . . I melted . . . I'd never seen such an expression. It was pure . . . and trusting and . . . and innocent; so . . . so guileless . . . an understanding so natural, so intense . . . an epiphany."

Then again, Albee taunts us, maybe the logic here is that Sylvia is an animal who becomes humanized because she is the object of unbridled human male sexuality. Albee is not saying this is what all males are like; he is playing with the common belief in his audience that this is what all males are like. What is debated in the play is whether cross-species rape is, from Martin's perspective, nonetheless a form of male sex. The play could not work were it not for that possibility: a man has sex with a farm animal. Far-fetched, but not entirely implausible. He is a man, after all.

Transgressive sex is not incidental or merely titillating in the play. The man-goat affair shocks because no words of affection or declarations of love can cover up the hideous vision of such an act of feral debauchery, just as images of Albee's carnal being forever agitated his own family, who responded to their gay son with censorious cruelty. As Albee has Martin insist, "I thought I was; I thought we *all* were . . . animals."

If men are just animals, it's not clear what counts as unnatural.[10]

FRISKY BONOBO APPETITES

Among the most popular science writers today we find a remarkable number of primatologists, whose research and insights into ape behavior have become legendary. When Koko the gorilla, who learned at least the rudiments of sign language, died, there were major obituaries in newspapers across the United States. (The degree to which Koko could actually communicate this way was always debated.) Jane Goodall and her chimpanzee studies have made her easily among the most recognized scientists in the world. Tales of gorillas and chimpanzees have such currency today for many reasons, but surely one of the most obvious is what we believe we are learning about ourselves.

For many of us who read about science for pleasure, psychologist and primatologist Frans de Waal and anthropologist and primatologist Sarah Blaffer Hrdy are favorite authorities on all things animal. Their focus has always been on nonhuman primates, and their most important discoveries have been based on careful observation of other kinds of animals and not their own. But the analysis each provides holds implications for us humans, including with respect to masculinity and femininity, violence and peace, and sexuality. Nonetheless, as de Waal has cautioned, and no doubt Hrdy would agree, "we also abuse nature by projecting our views onto it, after which we extract them again, circularly proving whatever view we hold."[11]

For centuries, we thought animals were entirely governed by unconscious instinct. But both de Waal and Hrdy have expanded our appreciation for animal choice and personality. In his many publications based on his work leading the Yerkes National Primate Research Center in Georgia, de Waal has repeatedly offered insights about where to draw the behavioral lines between animals, and how to develop our appreciation of how bendy those lines must be. Yerkes is one of seven national primate research centers funded by the US National Institutes of Health; it is located on 117 acres in Lawrenceville, Georgia, in rolling and wooded hills thirty miles northeast of Atlanta. When I visited in 2014, it housed over 2,000 nonhuman primates.

Arrival at the center feels like entering a military base, with all facilities fenced off, gates blocking entrances, signs warning not to take photos, and a security clearance checkpoint. Cameras and personnel monitor every movement on the grounds. De Waal meets visitors in an outbuilding with small offices and, alas, no distracting apes. Upon request, he sometimes allows them a quick observation from a position some distance from an internal fence separating off the chimpanzees.

De Waal has championed several enduring conceptual innovations based on his empirical work at Yerkes and elsewhere, among them his studies of bonobos, pygmy chimpanzees that share a common ancestor with the more common chimpanzees as well as humans. Merely 6 million years ago we were all one big happy species. Since then we have gone our largely separate ways, and one of the fascinating puzzles for primatologists is to figure out how these three species diverged. Often in his writings and interviews, de Waal chooses a particular trait he finds common to one or another ape and humans; through demonstrating similarities, he helps us to better appreciate the complex psychologies of apes.

With chimpanzees he has long railed against the mantra repeated in scientific and virtually every other quarter that chimpanzees are the closest evolutionary cousins to humans. De Waal believes that bonobos are just as close, but that we hear more about chimp cousinhood for reasons related to current beliefs about human males and females, sexuality, and violence rather than because of the actual evolutionary record. Chimpanzees spend more of their time than bonobos in aggressive activities ("Just like us!"); one common collective noun for a group of chimpanzees is "troop." Furthermore, their troops are in nearly all cases dominated by males ("Just like us!"). De Waal grows weary of colleagues drawing overly simplistic comparisons between chimps and humans, showing that often the aim is to "explain" that human male licentious sexuality and eruptions of violence are in some fashion ingrained, because you can find what looks like similar behavior among chimpanzees. The simple fact that male gorillas and chimpanzees have less interest in sex unless a female is fertile, for instance, seems a rather basic difference that would remove these ape relatives from close comparisons with humans, at least with respect to sexuality, the kind of point de Waal never tires of making.

Because bonobos are just as close to humans as chimpanzees are, de Waal's studies of them became especially important. Thanks to his research, we now know that bonobos have females in positions of high status, and that males and females spend a lot of their waking hours involved in sexual activities of wondrous kinds and combinations. This finding is directly relevant to humans because it shows a counterexample to chimpanzee male violence and alpha male social organization. The bonobos, in de Waal's words, "show that our lineage is marked not just by male dominance and xenophobia but also by a love of harmony and sensitivity to others."[12]

But here, too, we should be wary of looking too closely for human behavior. The fact that bonobos have sex with a range of individuals in their group, both same sex and opposite sex, whether or not the females are in estrus, distinguishes them not only from gorillas and chimpanzees but also from their human cousins. The fact is that humans, male as well as female, are far more picky about sexual partners than any of the other apes are.[13]

Throughout his many books and articles, de Waal seeks to make a middle run through the opposite poles of the same inanity: behavioralist scientists, for whom external stimuli ("conditioning") is everything and biology means little, and those who see animals as automatons doing little more than responding to internal stimuli. De Waal makes clear that one reason this should matter, for those of us not employed to watch monkeys fight, hump, emote, or console, has to do with the Nazis: "After World War II, I think people were very obsessed with aggressive behavior and violence. And actually, if you read the old books on evolution of humans, it's all about aggression. Everything was about violence and aggression, and all of the comparisons between humans and animals were on that front. There was a huge resistance to explaining human behavior biologically. It was equated with being a Nazi."[14]

By the time sociobiology came along in the mid-1970s, and especially by the 1990s, however, de Waal saw a shift to the point where

lectures on college campuses that explained sex differences in biological terms elicited yawns from students, who by then took all this for
granted. Yet biology for de Waal, in particular, does not mean adhering
to Victorian standards of gender and sexuality, or any other template in
which males and females are by nature endowed with conspicuously
distinct sexual appetites. And he is very much the historian of science
when he notes that male anthropologists especially have had "a lot of
trouble with the idea of female dominance much of the time among the
bonobo. I never heard a female primatologist or female anthropologist
tell me this is nonsense or this is not possible, or it's trivial."[15]

In addition to overturning gender refrains about what males and
females do and don't do across species, de Waal also doesn't like to talk
about innate biologies and instinct, because they cannot account for
much of what he has observed, from "chimpanzee politics" to primate
reconciliation, empathy, and emotions in general. Beyond tool use, de
Waal has written effectively about altruism, sexual orgasm, humor, cooperation, theory of mind, self-awareness, social reciprocity, and more
among our ape cousins.

He never shies away from delineating boundaries, such as communication ("I don't think apes have language") and fathering ("We are the
only animals . . . with the concept of paternity as a basis for fatherhood").
These are not trivial differences for him. But he doesn't particularly endorse the term "nonhuman animals," insisting that, as with Darwin, it's
all a matter of relatedness of animals of various kinds. De Waal's central
mission seems aimed at raising our human awareness and regard for the
fundamental capacities of other animals, especially those closest to us.[16]

"In relation to our close relatives," he told me, "I think there's nothing wrong with anthropomorphism, even though I would always add
that you still need to check if it is the same thing that you are seeing.
But if you get to very different species, let's say two octopi embrace each
other, that may not be the same sort of embrace as you will have as a
human being." Anthropomorphism works for de Waal, and he thinks it
should be more widely adopted by the rest of us.[17]

BANISHING COY FEMALES

Male apes are often seen as proxies for human males when they are believed to exhibit a pan-creature male attribute. But as with humans, you can learn a lot about male ape behavior by looking at female apes instead.

It is no accident that Sarah Blaffer Hrdy came along when she did in the 1970s, a time of heightened turmoil about gender and sexuality among humans, and revolutionized our understanding of female ape sexuality. She delivered a conceptual body-blow to long-held notions of sexual docility among female primates, and in so doing, in effect overturned long-established preconceptions about what distinguishes mammalian male and female sexual activity. The main purpose of her first pioneering work on langurs was not to gain insights into human females and males, but there can be no doubt that the feminist movement at the time was a background for her interests and findings. In addition, through Hrdy's primate studies we have been better able to recalibrate our underlying assumptions about male and female more broadly, leading to further clarity about mistaken assumptions, and perhaps not a little gender disorientation, too.

Squeezing facts to wedge them into preexisting theory can be a problem in any scientific field. Evolutionary psychologists are widely accused of selectively mining animal behavior for their models with the endgame purpose of showing some human activity as stamped with a Darwinian Seal of Evolutionary Approval. Sarah Hrdy is the exceptional sociobiologist who has been willing to rethink hallowed truths based on new evidence. And as she would be the first to note, the fact that she is a woman and that most of her major discoveries have to do with female primates is entirely to the point. Before Hrdy, few if any scientists studied female primates with as much care and open-mindedness.

In reconceiving several basic beliefs about female primate behavior, Hrdy has rewritten the book on mothering, allomothering (when other females help in parenting), infanticide, primate sexuality (including with

respect to female coyness, sexual assertiveness, polyandry, and promis-
cuity), and sexism in the sciences.

Consider the following numbers that come from observations of
others but in Hrdy's hands take on new meanings: a female chimpanzee
may well have 6,000 copulations with dozens of males in the course of
her life and give birth to five offspring. Standard-issue biology courses
teach that males are profligate and females modest and choosy. Hrdy
demolished the notion of the textbook coy female, showing that, in case
after case, when anyone (i.e., female primatologists) bothered to look,
lo and behold, plenty of female primates were scampering around and
copulating even when, god forbid, they were not in estrus. Maybe they
liked sex?[18]

In studying langurs and libido, Hrdy admits that it has been hard
to restrain the urge to extrapolate to our species: "Once acquired, the
habit of comparing humans with other primates is hard to shake."
When I mentioned to her that Frans de Waal had said something similar to me, she chuckled and replied, "I refer to him as my only adult
colleague."[19]

Yet she is comfortable delineating between humans and animals.
"Across cultures and between individuals, more variation exists [among
humans] in the form and extent of paternal investment than in all
other primates combined." As for paternity, and whether human males
ever know for sure who their offspring are—long "an obsessive focus
for evolutionary interpretations of male behavior"—for Hrdy, paternity
uncertainty "is only one factor influencing men's nurturing responses
to babies."[20]

The key is to test, and when necessary to disprove, existing presumptions about primates. Many of the beliefs she ended up dislodging
had to do with an overly dichotomous model in which female primates
(including female humans) were sexually demure, and male primates
had an insatiable craving to mate with as many females as they possibly could. According to Rebecca Jordan-Young, a multidisciplinary researcher who studies the science of sex differences, the male-as-predator,

female-as-passive-receptacle template prevailed in studies of sexuality until the 1980s: it was not simply that male and female were distinct, but that they were seen as polar opposites, a model in which female sexuality "followed a sort of romantic, sleeping-beauty model."[21]

Sarah Hrdy overturned implicit assumptions that female behavior boiled down to maternal behavior, and therefore, among other things, that sex could not be an end in itself for female primates. Her peers had long intoned "only hundreds of eggs, but billions of sperm . . . hundreds of eggs, but billions of sperm," as if these numbers in themselves proved that males as a group are sexually voracious—that they could afford to "waste" sperm, whereas females had to be sexually judicious to make every one of their precious ova count.[22]

One of Hrdy's early studies was especially poorly received by both certain feminists and sociobiologists. Based on her own work in the 1970s with langurs in southern India, she came to the then-astonishing conclusion that polyandrous mating by females was more widespread than had been understood, and for some primates it was downright normal. The feminist concern was that Hrdy linked biology too closely with sexuality. The sociobiologists expressed alarm because this notion challenged some basic premises of their evolutionary theory: polyandrous females simply did not fit with the dominant existing theory that (1) females need male provisioning, (2) if females were to engage in multiple couplings with many males they would risk forfeiting this male commitment, so that (3) males may couple widely but females have an inbuilt incentive to be more selective. The implications for female *and* male primate sexuality were shocking.[23]

The cherry on the top of this revisionist sundae was the extension of Hrdy's analysis from the apes to humans, and speculation about the origins of "patrilineal interests" among humans. Prior to the Neolithic (roughly 10,000 BC), Hrdy believes, "women would be most likely to mate polyandrously with several men where support from matrilineal kin (including help provisioning young) provided them the social leverage to do so."[24]

Combine that with the tantalizing theories about female sexuality recently advanced by ornithologist Richard Prum on the evolution of beauty—"Because the female orgasm has evolved through a purely aesthetic evolutionary process of mate choice, women actually *do* have the capacity for greater sexual pleasure than men, and women's sexual pleasure *is* more expansive in quality as well as extent"—and you have all the fixings for a radical new appreciation for the capacity of not just our bonobo cousins, and not just our males, for lifelong, lively sexual encounters.[25]

ANTHROPOMORPHISTS GONE WILD

How do we know when we're pushing animal comparisons too far?

For most of us, everyday anthropomorphism centers on the attention we lavish worldwide on our 600 million cats and 500 million dogs, under observation and interacting with us round the clock, those pets with human names and personalities. Nonhuman animals may be humanized: treated as sharing basic qualities like sentience and volition, as having more of an individual mind than a pack mentality, and sometimes even as possessing consciousness, in the sense of having memory of the past and expectations for the future. Nonhuman animals are anthropomorphized so that they can be elevated. When humans become animalized, however, they are in effect dehumanized and degraded. They lose their singular qualities. They are thought to surrender to herd impulse. They lose much of their self-control and ability to choose.

It is not easy to find the borders between acceptable and insupportable anthropomorphism. Where do we draw the lines, especially when thinking about men as animals? Notre Dame primatologist Agustín Fuentes offers a clue: "It's a commonly held belief that if you strip away culture, that which keeps us well behaved, then a beastly savage will emerge (especially in men)." The closer we get to the idea of men as animals who cannot control themselves but need to be kept in line, the more we should exercise care in our language and presumptions.[26]

Anthropomorphism among paleoanthropologists—whose attention is keyed to ancestors who knuckle-scraped the earth millions of years ago—logically enough often focuses on how close in time we are to a shared ancestor. We parted ways with the ancestors of orangutans 14 million years ago. With gorilla-human progenitors, it was 8 million years ago. And as we know, as to the foreparents we share with chimpanzees and bonobos, the fork in the evolutionary road was as recent as 6 million years ago. Almost by definition, we must therefore share more habits of heart, mind, and genitalia with chimps than gorillas, more with gorillas than orangs. The closer in this scale of time, the more the same nouns and verbs are used to describe our respective behaviors.

Look at the many terms listed in Table 2 that are employed widely by zoologists and primatologists to describe nonhuman animals. Take your time decoding and considering which ones seem most reasonable and which are too laden with uniquely human stamps to be usefully applied to other animals. (Hint: specialists debate the utility of employing these terms all the time.) Put an "A" (for appropriate) or an "I" (for inappropriate) next to each one.

Some Anthropomorphic Terms Commonly Used by Scientists

Adolescent male risk-taking	Feeling
Aggression	Fight
Agriculture	Harem
Alliance	Infidelity
Anger	Kidnapping
Bonding	Maternal instinct
Caste	Matrilineal social organization
Courtship	Play
Crushes	Polygyny
Cultural innovation	Prostitution
Culture	Queen
Dalliance	Rape, rapist
Despot	Slavery, slave
Displaced aggression	Taxes/investments/costs/benefits
Dominance	Torture
Family chauvinism	War
Fear	

Why you put an "A" or an "I" is the question. If "anger" seemed to you to work across the species board, why not "slavery"? If "alliance" seemed like an appropriate way to characterize marauding hordes of monkeys, then why not call the ensuing conflict an example of monkey "war"? We hear these terms used, and we use them ourselves, and rarely think twice about the implications of drawing such tight parallels between the actions and feelings of nonhuman animals and our own behavior and emotions.

No one really expects that nonhuman animals use speech to converse, but anthropomorphic talking animals are always popular—and at least for the genus of Equus they can trace their ancestry back to biblical times. In Numbers 22:28–30, we read, "And the LORD opened the mouth of the ass, and she said unto Balaam, What have I done unto thee, that thou hast smitten me these three times? And Balaam said unto the ass, Because thou hast mocked me: I would there were a sword in mine hand, for now would I kill thee. And the ass said unto Balaam, Am not I thine ass, upon which thou hast ridden ever since I was thine unto this day? was I ever wont to do so unto thee? and he said, Nay." It took the miracle of a talking donkey to get through Balaam's thick skull that the Lord wanted him to wake up and find the righteous path.[27]

Every primatologist uses certain of these human categories to describe the behavior of nonhuman species. The vocabulary most readily at hand is what is used to describe human relationships and acts, and many try hard to find apt replacements for words that crudely anthropomorphize animal behavior. Anthropomorphic terms can seem applicable—"Those male monkeys are fighting." They can be a playful way to compare nonhuman animals to humans—"That female monkey is presenting to that male." And they can be a fabulous way to gain insight and sympathy for animals—"That female monkey is a good mother." Perhaps we should leave it there. If we've learned anything in the past few decades it is that nonhuman animals have far more varied and rich lives emotionally, organizationally, and sexually than we ever realized.

In order to think more critically about anthropomorphism we need to allow for the foundational reality of evolution and our common origins as well as for the (just as real) abuse of human-animal comparisons. These comparisons often reveal more about social and cultural bias than they do about similar cross-species' motives or meanings. This will become clearer if we take a closer look at three recurrent, contemporary examples of what can happen when anthropomorphism is given free rein. These examples demonstrate how three terms in particular, first built on flawed notions of male and female sexuality as polar opposites, serve to reinforce these mistaken preconceptions. They are hummingbird *prostitutes*, baboon *harems*, and mallard duck *gang rape*.[28]

Prostitution in this case is a way to talk about female hummingbirds "offering" the male hummingbirds sexual congress in exchange for something else—twigs for a nest, for example. Offering what certain ornithologists regard as the female hummingbird point of view, hummingbird sex appears transactional, and that seems (to certain birdbrained scientists) the essence of human prostitution. The unstated premise is that males and females (hummingbird and human alike) have sex for dissimilar reasons, which for the females is to get something besides sex. The parallel between hummingbird and human affects how we understand hummingbird behavior, and more importantly, for our purposes, also reinforces the idea that there is something natural (and maybe, therefore, necessary) about human prostitution, and that females of both species have sex for reasons other than sexual pleasure.

The term "harem" is used even more widely among scientists, to describe a scene in which single males—for example, baboons—have sex with many different females, which is, at best, an American teenage boy's interpretation of a harem. I have yet to see one primatologist use the term "harem" with so much as a sentence defining what he means by harem, much less an inkling of an informed description or a semblance of an analysis of the shape, texture, rationale, history, and lived experience of any human harems.

In one account after another of mallard duck behavior, the term "rape" is applied with relative shamelessness. Sometimes we read about "forced copulation," which is a step in the right direction. But even there, given that human rape could also be called forced copulation, we remain in semantic quicksand. Groups of male mallard ducks do coordinate what we can call attacks on single females, with the end event of a male copulating with the female duck. Male mallards engage in such attacks as part of routine behavior that impregnates the female. Of significance, however, ornithologist Richard Prum reports, "In several duck species, including Mallards, in which the forced copulations are a stunning 40 percent of the total copulations, *only 2–5 percent* of the young in the nest are sired by a male who is not the chosen partner of the female. Thus, the overwhelming number of forced copulations are unsuccessful."[29]

Male mallards do not attack female ducklings in this way. They do not attack other males in this way. And crucially, if you follow a male mallard duck, you will be witness to this kind of behavior nearly half the time. In what world could you say the same about any human male you know? There may be some male mallards who are more successful than others with these attacks, but there are none for whom this is abhorrent behavior. Thus, to equate the actions of mallard ducks with human gang rape requires us to see rape as fundamentally instinctual for males across species, and to understand a human woman's consent (or lack thereof) as fundamentally equivalent to a duck's.

If challenged, those who use these terms often admit they are meant to be memorable more than precise. It's true that exaggeration, surprise, and analogies are all useful instructional tools. But relying on them to this extent has taught us to overidentify with particular animal behaviors and then implicate instinct or nature as the source of individual and culture-specific human activities. When psychologist Steven Pinker writes that "infidelity is common even in so-called pair-bonded species," we just have to ask: If infidelity is premised on marriage vows, then when did the invitations go out for those weddings? The fact is that

Pinker or I can be party to infidelity, but the swans on the Charles River cannot, any more than can prairie voles or shingleback skinks in their habitats. Infidelity is a uniquely *human* experience. To call swan sex with more than one mate infidelity obscures what and why swans do this, and more importantly, it naturalizes human adultery beyond reach.[30]

Among the many omissions in each of these cases of anthropomorphism is that with virtually every behavior, human males and females show more variation than has been observed among males and females in any other species. So while it is entirely predictable that a male mallard duck, for involuntary reasons of reproduction, will engage in what some call gang rape, this is absolutely not the case for human males, where rape is a matter of social power and prerogative. Even when gang rape occurs during wartime, it is not the biological maleness of the rapists that causes it. To call what mallard ducks do gang rape has real consequences undoubtedly beyond those intended, because this language can inadvertently lend seeming biological support for gang rape among humans.

Rarely does a researcher compare humans and animals in an all-inclusive manner. No one says that human males are entirely like chimpanzee males. Rather, particular traits are selectively employed to bolster a larger contention. To be sure, we share a common ancestry, and our DNA is remarkably similar to that of chimpanzees. But if that's all it takes to make meaningful comparisons, we might also note that human DNA is 35 percent similar to that of daffodils, which really gets us nowhere.[31]

ANTHROPODENIAL

The flip side of extreme anthropomorphism is what Frans de Waal calls *anthropodenial,* a term he defines as "the a priori rejection of shared characteristics between humans and animals when in fact they may exist." If your main concern is an underappreciation of animals and their emotional complexity, you may bend the stick more in the direction of warning against rejecting common patterns. If your main concern is human gender relations, however, it is not hard to see that overdone comparisons can lead to a different set of problems clustered around the notion that human males behave more in sync with one another than is the case, and are compelled by their bodies, not decision making, to do things like committing rape. Human rape is a choice, not an accident or a hardwired compulsion.[32]

It has not been just humans that continued to evolve over the past several million years. De Waal writes, "People often think that the apes must have stood still while we evolved, but genetic data in fact suggests that chimpanzees changed *more* than we did." So looking at chimps and bonobos as somehow illustrative of what "we" all were millions of years ago is deeply flawed. For de Waal, "the key point is that anthropomorphism is not always as problematic as people think. To rail against it for the sake of scientific objectivity often hides a pre-Darwinian mindset, one uncomfortable with the notion of humans as animals." He is talking about creationists, and his point is watertight.[33]

The rub is that even for people who have no problem acknowledging that humans are animals, anthropomorphism can have negative effects, and it's good to be wary of some of them. If I mention to a queen ant that I admire her majestic ways, she will not know the difference. I can call her anything I like and it will not affect her in any way. But if I talk to my barber about slavery among ants, tell him that slavery is something that is found cross-species, that it's actually not uncommon, that human slavery is not the exception but almost the rule in the animal kingdom, it could sound like I am saying something fundamental about human beings, too. I could leave my barber with the impression that slavery is natural, and therefore, as awful as it is, pretty much impossible to ever eradicate from human societies, just as it is impossible to eradicate it from ant societies. The words we use and the meanings behind them influence how we understand human relationships and events. They can cause trauma—to people, not ants—for generations after slavery.[34]

Humans have their uniqueness, and they have their *Umwelt*, their animal point of view and particularity, and we need to appreciate that. Talking about slavery among other species can do more than trivialize human oppression; it can spread ideas that support it. If people learn about a coming hurricane, this does not change their beliefs about the weather patterns that caused the storm. But if they hear about "slavery" among ants, could this not change their beliefs about what has given rise to slavery among humans?

It is one thing to insist that we extend to other animals features that previously were held to be uniquely human—in a sense, to humanize the animals. Anthropomorphism can be lighthearted and a mnemonic device to make sense of the world. But we need to be precise. As one who studies the human species, I feel it is particularly salient to humans (and their core cognitive abilities) how we characterize them and their affinities to other species. It doesn't mean that we can't or shouldn't find continuities and parallels. It does mean that psychological and socio-logical profiling can have a lasting impact on humans. De Waal quotes Mark Twain: "Man is the only animal that blushes—or needs to."[35]

And, speaking of blushing, that is a quintessential experience that is highly gendered (and racialized) among humans. In the English-speaking world, white women blush. White men turn red. And that, too, speaks volumes about anthropomorphism, because nowhere does it have more impact than in making analogies about male and female among different species. When metaphor and analogy make human activities like harems and infidelity look "natural" because they are said to appear throughout the animal kingdom, we fall into the trap primatologist Stephen Jay Gould warned against:

> Metaphor is a dangerous, if ineluctable, device. We use images and analogies to foster understanding of complex and unfamiliar sub-jects, but we run the risk of falsely infusing nature with the baggage of our parochial prejudices or idiosyncratic social arrangements. The situation can become truly insidious, even perversely so (in the

literal rather than pejorative sense), when we impose a human institution upon nature by false metaphor—and then try to justify the
social phenomenon as an inevitable reflection of nature's dictates![36]

I teach a course on gender and science and use the examples of
hummingbirds, baboons, and mallard ducks to discuss their relevance
for human gender relations. I ask the students if evolutionary overrides
could apply to humans as well. Discussion is always lively, and there
is rarely uniform agreement. One year, a week after this lecture about
applying the labels for complicated, historically grounded human relationships to nonhuman animal behaviors, a young woman came to
class and shocked us. She had in the interim attended a biology class
in which her professor had instructed the students on the workings of
"gangbanging bacteria." You decide: witty or warped?[37]

Anthropomorphism might make the study of nonhuman animals,
or bacteria, more user-friendly and easier to understand. Except if you
happen to be a person who has been the target of a very human gang
rape—or any other assault, for that matter. Why take these clever and
transparently over-the-top comparisons so seriously? For so many reasons,
not the least of which is the normalization of rape as a part of nature. You
can joke this way to a bacterium all you want, calling it a gangbanger or
anything else, and I would wager my tenure that the bacterium will not
be offended. Talk of rape and its ubiquity among human organisms in
this way, however, and listeners can draw lessons that are nothing short
of felonious.

When scientists uncritically anthropomorphize not just about other
animal species but even single-celled organisms, it is hard to know
whether to be outraged, or just relieved that the comparison is so outlandish that no one could take it seriously. We can find plenty of evidence that discussion about what is naturally male across animal species
has always been prominent in otherwise very different societies. Aristotle
memorably wrote on zoology; before Aristotle, Confucius contemplated
the relationship between humans and other animals. But an emphasis

on men's animality has particular consequences and potency today. We are at a crucial moment in gender history, one in which we need to get better at broadening our definitions about what it means to be a man.

Too often, anthropomorphism has served other animals better than it has served humans. If our aim is to appreciate the range of qualities our primate cousins embody and express, and that there are indeed profound and abundant similarities between chimps, bonobos, and humans, point well taken. But if the aim is to use human relationships to characterize nonhuman ones, and then turn this back to imply that because these are shared traits they will always be with us (or with us until evolved out), that's not just careless anthropomorphism, it's ape abuse.

Here's the crux of the matter: we should never lose sight of the critical fact that all animals vary in their behaviors, and that human males are exquisitely malleable, having a range of behavior markedly greater than those of the males of any other species. Humans don't have to act like other animals. Believing that we do is reckless. To lose sight of human mutability and the range of behavior among humans is to give men a morphological free pass to tyrannize others under the guise of "acting like a guy," and to offer men the impunity of evolutionary inheritance for a defense.

CHAPTER FOUR

THE MALE LIBIDO

I think about sex, therefore I am.
Ralph Messenger, in *Thinks . . .*, DAVID LODGE

WHEN WE THINK ABOUT SEXUAL SELECTION, SEXUAL ENTITLE-ment, and sexual choices, why are we so vulnerable to precon-ceptions about differences between men's and women's sexualities? A lot of these notions are rooted in the gender binary that has been coming under fire in recent years. Despite the "rediscovery" of fe-male sexual pleasure in the 1960s and 1970s—truly one of the great social accomplishments of the late twentieth century—there are few areas of human activity that are more bifurcated in our thinking than sexuality. Our double vision on male-versus-female sexuality will remain in place as long as we resist a similar reassessment of male libido. Otherwise we are faced with enduring myths about men and sex, hallowed scientific certainties about maleness and mascu-linity, and, in the continued facile glorification of male sexuality, what amounts to a social bias that prevents serious reconsideration of masculinities.

IVY LEAGUE SEXUAL SELECTION

A good place to start looking at the overexamined but under-understood topic of men and sex is Brown University, where I teach. And, sorry, but don't get your hopes up of salacious tales of the now-defunct annual "Sex Power God" LGBTQ-sponsored party at Brown that made headlines for its reputedly rampant nudity and sex.

There is a biology course at Brown that has featured a set of slides for a particular lecture. Over the years, students have sent me copies of these slides. Made to support a lecture on sexual selection, it has included slides of rams butting horns, peacocks strutting for peahens, and insects, reptiles, and birds all with the same pattern: the males fighting each other, with the fittest males getting first dibs on sex with females. Meanwhile, coy and fussy as always, the females selected only those males they deemed to be the fittest fathers for their future offspring. Take home message: when it came to sex, males of all species were pretty much the same.

The lesson was not so different from that of the nature shows many of the students grew up on. But then came the punchline, delivered in the form of more slides, including one of football players (male, of course, in uniform on the field) and cheerleaders (all female, of course, in uniform, on the sidelines), with text on the left side of the slide that read:

- Males should be competitive
  » Fight for additional mates
- Females should be "choosy"
  » Allocate their expensive resources efficiently

You see, students, we're all remarkably similar when it comes to sexual selection and the process through which males and females of every species, including the human, hook up with one another. Males display for the females, females select males. These slides were aimed precisely at an audience working overtime to figure out their own sexualities, and the implication was that males were a horde of self-fluffers, seeking to procreate indiscriminately, and females were picky about sexual partners.

Leaving aside for now the suspect contention of evolutionary biologists that it is entirely reasonable to compare the mating habits of pipefish, beetles, rhinoceroses, and humans, what are we to make of sexual selection, the twin key concept to Charles Darwin's theory of natural selection? Sexual selection is the concept that tries to explain the significance of everything from sexual dimorphism (differences in average body size for males and females) to parental investment in offspring and female fussiness, also known as "the limiting factor." It is easy to grow inured to thinking about humans in terms of two genders. Yet far from something static, as neuroscientist Lise Eliot insists, "gender differences are a moving target."[1]

The biological binaries are now routine: females are limited by the number of eggs they produce, whereas males produce more sperm than they can handle. Males are larger in size, which for witless wombats just as much as Mar-a-Lago plutocrats is held to correlate with males contesting over females: only the natural "weaponry" of the males differs, whether that be claws or forked tongues. In the Brown biology class lecture, photos of male and female caribou, flies, newts, sticklebacks, and frigatebirds were used to illustrate the pugnacious and the coquettish—you don't need to take the class to guess which is male and which female. Yet by far the most startling and disheartening of the images—shown in the middle of all these other animal shots, and accompanied by the professor's biological explanations for commonalities across the animal, marine, and insect kingdoms—were the ones highlighting football players and cheerleaders. In what amounted to a test of quasi-religious faith, the students were in a sense implored to rise up in a spiritual reckoning to accept the truth: sex distinguishes, sex unites, and sex manipulates all creatures large and small.[2]

You can practically hear the males of all species shouting: "Yes to sex with her. Yes with her. Yes with her. Yes with her. Well, only maybe with her. Yes with her. Yes with her. Well, OBVIOUSLY, yes with her!"

Meanwhile, the finicky females are responding: "No to sex with him. No with him. No with him. No with him. Well, maybe with him. No with him. No with him. Well, FINALLY, yes with him!"

Not surprisingly, these views of male and female sexuality mapped perfectly onto existing stereotypes in the United States about such matters. But what would be made of the belief reported in Andalusia, Spain, that women are seductresses whose sexual appetites are more insatiable and lustful than men's, or that women in Morocco are considered more sexually rapacious than men, or that the Dani of Indonesia have historically practiced a four-to-six-*year* postpartum sexual abstinence for men and women?[3]

The science of maleness can reinforce prejudices and give way to acquiescent resignation that some things sexual are too ingrained to change. That conclusion is as bad for young men as for young women, because it lends credence to male sexual aggression, enshrines female fastidiousness, and with that reinforces patriarchal ideas about sexuality, specifically consent.

WATCHING PORN IN THE MALE BRAIN

Having a little knowledge may be a dangerous thing. But having and disseminating a lot of erroneous knowledge about men and sex can be far more dangerous. And intentions be damned: the road to hell is paved with the faulty findings of expert wisdom on men's sexuality. This is a story about pornography, or, more precisely, men watching porn. It was sparked, improbably enough, during a job interview.

For reasons that will become clear, keep in mind that the year was 1996. After my job talk earlier in the day, I made sure to arrive early for the all-important job dinner. The chair of the search committee was already at the restaurant, sitting at the bar. I sat down next to him. The department was known for its strengths in the field of psychological anthropology, and I was now sitting with the grand poohbah himself. He was a fierce advocate for the science of cognition and behavior, including gender, sex, and sexuality. That men and women in many, if not all, matters represented polar opposites in cognition and behavior was for him a given. His favorite intellectual sparring partners were the cultural relativists, who challenged his views as crude generalizations.

Over drinks, as we waited for the others in the party to arrive, he steered the discussion toward gender. He introduced a line of reasoning about what is naturally gendered, and therefore unresponsive to cultural influence, and which gender differences are more varied across cultures, and therefore potentially responsive to cultural change. He offered what he considered to be a gold-standard example of biological differences that divided all men from all women: visual cues. Men were visual thinkers, hardwired in such a way to be visually stimulated more than women, for instance, when it came to pornography. Didn't I agree that the overwhelming number of viewers of porn were men? In 1996, I had to admit it seemed that way. Well, then, how else could I explain this except through something built into men's physical selves? That was my challenge, and I didn't, and perhaps couldn't, meet it well that day.

I did counter that I didn't think this was true. My proof? Frankly, I was weak on the evidentiary side of the conversation. I insisted that women and men were not so different when it came to sexual stimulation and visual prompts. Where were the studies to back up what I was claiming when it came to visual stimulation? He had plenty. I didn't have any. I had a gut feeling I was correct, though of course I could not respond with such a claim.[4]

Around this time, in the mid-1990s, the Internet was taking off and porn with it. All you needed was a credit card to sample an all-you-can-watch buffet of videos from the privacy of your home. Little did the committee chair or I realize that within a few short years, porn viewership by women as well as men would grow to a multibillion-dollar industry. It was not a good move to contradict the head of the search committee, I will grant you, and I was not an expert in the realm of cognitive studies of visual or any other cues. But as it turned out, I was right.

We need to be especially wary of studies that confirm social ste-reotypes about gender. As we have seen, the science of masculinity is shot through with bias, and it can seep into even the most specialized, objective-sounding pronouncements and cloud our understanding about men and maleness. The more specialized the scientific knowl-edge in question, the harder it becomes to question it. It's easy to weigh in on topics like visual stimulation. Brain circuitry can seem beyond comprehension for most of us. But based on the precedents, there is good reason to not always believe everything you're told by experts.

When we compare brains in boys and girls, we find two notable dif-ferences: boys' brains are, on average, slightly (8–10 percent) larger than girls' brains, and girls' brains tend to finish growing a year or two before boys' brains. That's it. Yet the reality that male and female brains start off essentially the same has somehow escaped the attention of the media and broader public. It can be more appealing to emphasize differences between the sexes, and to trace differences back not just puckishly to gender planets of origin, but to material, unvarying, and unalterable features of biology, such as brain types. But talk of gendered brain types, my third example of biased examples about absolute male-female gen-der differences, is driven by ideology. It is not good science.[5]

The biological anthropologist Richard Bribiescas believes that boys and girls behave differently because of cultural and social influences, but that biological sex-based distinctions do exist. He writes, "It would be naive to assume that millions of years of mammalian evolution in-volving differential selection pressures on males and females would result in a single brain type that is not selected to deal with sex-specific challenges."[6]

Beyond the conflation of sex and gender here, even if we grant that it makes no sense that millions of years of mammalian evolution gives us a single brain type, we do not necessarily arrive at the thesis that therefore we have two brain types and only two, and that these two co-incide with two types of sex organs, and not by accident. This idea can appeal to commonsense experience about differences between men and women. But those differences have to hold for all times and all places, and they simply don't. Historical and cultural variation make an entire mess of such neat, biological distinctions.

"We love this stuff," writes Lise Eliot. "It's fun to be different. It makes romance more exciting and provides endless fodder for late-night comedians. *But there's enormous danger in this exaggeration of sex differences*, first and foremost in the expectations it creates among parents, teachers, and children themselves." She goes on to alert us that when we dwell on differences perceived to be natural, differences that are not in fact rooted in brain biology, we can raise our children with reinforced if specious stereotypes about boys and girls.[7]

There are several problems with dividing brains into male and female ones. First, even defining male and female biologically has proved more difficult than this framework would allow. Chromosomes don't always paint a clear picture. Or hormone levels—within a wide range of normal levels, androgens and estrogens are not predictive of any particular behavior in men or women. Or sex organs—more people have part-male, part-female genitals than is often acknowledged. More importantly, we can easily exaggerate the differences that do exist. Even if most people have largely similar one-or-the-other apparatuses, appearances can be deceiving, as Anne Fausto-Sterling showed in a series of biological studies on intersexed people. Fausto-Sterling listed several types of intersexuality beyond ambiguous genitalia, including Turner syndrome (where females lack a second X chromosome), Klinefelter syndrome (where males have an extra X chromosome), androgen insensitivity syndrome (a genetically inherited change in the cell's surface receptor for testosterone), and more. Most of all, Fausto-Sterling advises against pinning sex and sexuality and everything that goes with them on the form of someone's genitals.[8]

If that's true of gonads, why should it be otherwise with brains?

Some of those who posit an underlying premise linking brains and genitals trace the reasons back hundreds of thousands of years to human evolution and the emergence of a standard and universal division of labor between males and females. Men went hunting game, while women raised the babies and gathered nuts and berries. Over time, the males who were more aggressive and self-sufficient were more successful hunters than the less aggressive, less self-sufficient males, and therefore these traits among men were selected for through evolutionary pressures. Tasked with raising the young, the evolutionary pressure on females over time was to select for more nurturant qualities.

If such qualities were so mutually exclusive and restricted to either men or women, this argument might even make sense. But what happened to women who lost male mates? Did they automatically have to look for other males? Or could they themselves take up hunting? The answers are so obvious it pains me to have to report that some women who lost mates found other ones, some did not, some did fine, some did not, and success did not in itself depend on finding a mate. What is more, there is ample evidence in the archaeological record that until about 15,000 years ago hunting was a far more communal, male *and* female activity than was true later as animals became more scarce.

Contemporary arguments about men and women positing limits for women in math, leadership, and combat—and disparaging men for their lack of ability in child-rearing and emotional expression, as well as for their propensity to be risk-takers—often assume these qualities are built in, and based in evolution. Ultimately, they are grounded in beliefs about men's and women's brains being significantly dissimilar because of their distinctive privates. But even if we grant that there are two major types of brains, why this bifurcation exists, and why it would reflect male-female divisions of labor, and not, say, height, weight, or 20/20 vision—all factors that could conceivably impinge on how one operates in the world—may reveal more about presuppositions than it does about scientific fact and evolution. It has to do with preconceived notions of male and female characteristics.

Neuroscientist Daphna Joel agrees, maintaining that although sex differences in brain structure are well documented, in terms of both size and composition, thinking of brains as party to human sexual dimorphism is incorrect. Instead of thinking of brains as taking only one of two forms, male or female, we would do better to think of brains as intersexed, a "heterogeneous mosaic" that "can take different forms that are not aligned on a continuum between a 'male brain' and a 'female brain.'"[9]

Differences in brain types by sex begin in utero: for boys-in-the-making, there is a surge in testosterone six weeks after conception and up to the end of the second trimester of pregnancy. But we should not take this information and draw flawed assumptions from it that imply a one-directional causal connection between biology and behavior later on, and, more specifically, a binary biology that provides a template restricting all human activity. What this perspective leaves out is the possibility of behavior changing brains, of environment seriously affecting biology, and of the brain as being more malleable than recalcitrant. This point about malleability is especially relevant for understanding perhaps the most important insight of recent neuroscience: whatever differences in brain chemistry and circuitry have been found between men and women, they were found, indeed, between men and women, that is, adult humans. Among children these differences are far less apparent, meaning that decades of cultural and social interactions along the gender binary can literally remodel brains along more sex-based lines.

If we simply step back and examine just the historical record from Europe, the myopia of the present moment becomes clearer. And not just Europe, but ancient Europe. What seems timeless and universal today in an ahistorical, prelapsarian cosmology about sex, brains, men, and women has changed in remarkable ways throughout history. If we traveled back millennia to the age of Jupiter, the Roman King of the Gods, we would certainly learn what everyone then knew to be the case: like it or not, women's libido and sexual pleasure was greater than men's. That's just the way it was. Time-traveling forward until we reached the early modern era, in about 1600, we would learn for a fact that despite superficial appearances, women and men had identical genitalia; the sole difference was that men's were outies and women's were innies. Coming forward still further, to about two hundred years ago, we could witness the invention by doctors of the science of two sexes, and the subsequent deposing of us all from a happier sexual perch of shared enjoyment to a time when, in the words of Berkeley historian Thomas Laqueur, "female orgasm . . . was banished to the borderlands of physiology."[10]

Neuroscience provides ample evidence of the brain's malleable capacity, of greater brain differences between men and between women than between men and women, and of the astounding sex brain differences that emerge not from conception but only after childhood. Despite parents' beliefs about their sons and daughters being from different planets, "overall, boys' and girls' brains are remarkably alike," writes Lise Eliot. But because "your brain is what you do with it," learning and practice rewire it. Which is why she concludes that "it would be shocking if the two sexes' brains *didn't* work differently by the time they were adults."[11]

In one classic study, Janet Hyde found in 2015 that of 124 psychological traits, including attributes long held to be sacrosanct exemplars of gender differences—mathematics performance, verbal ability, aggressive behavior, and moral reasoning—78 percent of the differences were small or close to zero. Hyde concludes, "It is time to consider the costs of overinflated claims of gender difference." It is our ideas about sex and gendered brains that can be truly limiting. The newer biological fields of epigenetics and gene transfer point the way to far more fundamental interactionism between genes and environment than we have previously acknowledged, as we will see in Chapter 9, but even they cannot by themselves unseat or erase prejudices about men and women and sexuality.[12]

MEN ARE ANIMAL SEX

The anthropologist Lourdes Arizpe has declared that "the spread of contraception has ruptured the previously existing physiological fatalism."

That goes for her native Mexico and every other country on earth. Until the early 1970s, Mexico had what is known in the population business as a pronatalist policy: keep those babies coming, the more the merrier, because, government authorities believed, greater population meant more labor power, and a bigger workforce meant greater economic and political clout in the hemisphere and across the globe. Demographers in Mexico had been trying to prevail on federal and state strategic planners, warning of too many youths coming of age and facing too few job prospects, but as in many impoverished countries throughout the 1960s, the unanimous mantra of Mexican officials was: POPULATION GROWTH = PROGRESS![13]

Then a remarkable change occurred, and government policy wonks did a quick about-face between 1972 and 1974: they came to fully support efforts to promote family planning, making contraceptives as widely available as possible.

Robert McNamara, then head of the World Bank, was a strong proponent of such moves, insisting that, "to put it simply: the greatest single obstacle to the economic and social advancement of the majority of peoples in the underdeveloped world is rampant population growth." Mexico's demographers had finally convinced the Mexican government to change course and end its population growth policies, but it took decades for the new policies to be implemented throughout the nation. Eventually, Mexico's birthrate fell from around six or seven children per woman to a little over two, on average. One can neatly map the spread of the birth control measures, beginning in the middle-class sectors of large cities, then expanding out through the slums of these same metropoles, into medium-sized cities, and across the countryside. By the 1990s, even the most remote hamlets of Oaxaca had visits from government public health personnel or nurses supported by Mexfam, an International Planned Parenthood Federation affiliate.[14]

Then a not-so-remarkable change happened. Or, rather, an adaptation on an old pattern. It was so inconspicuous and commonsensical, and unintentional, that there was no controversy. To most people the change went unnoticed and did not seem like a change at all: men were planned out of family planning. This happened less through the explicit exclusion of men and more by simply ignoring men in new family planning campaigns. It should come as no surprise that the emphasis was and had to be on women's reproductive health and sexuality. According to every social index, women were less well served in the public health sector than men; the government and every national and international funding agency recognized this and took steps to remedy the intolerable situation.

As soon as modern, relatively safe and reliable methods of birth control became available to them, the vast majority of Mexican women who wanted to prevent pregnancy adopted birth control pills, IUDs, and later, injectables and tubal ligations. The logic of women taking responsibility for family planning was levelheaded and laudable, and no one playing a significant role in promoting birth prevention—neither government health institutions, nor Mexfam, nor the international foundations supporting the work, such as Ford and Rockefeller— questioned whether and how men should be included in these new efforts. Men do not get pregnant. Men have fewer sexual and reproductive health issues. Men simply have different sexual and reproductive biologies. And women were in the most dire need of assistance in every aspect of their health, including around reproduction. There are some problems associated with planning men out of family planning, however, and the biggest one is that you cannot hope to achieve anything approaching gender equality if you exclude men from the discussion and decision making around the use of contraception. You also create a self-fulfilling prophecy if you discount men by establishing programs based on the idea that men are not interested in limiting the number of their offspring, timing the births of their children, caring for the women with whom they have children, or being a good father in these and other ways.

Leaving aside what many could more easily see as cultural issues of women shouldering the bulk of child care and parenting, women's

particular and pressing sexual and reproductive needs were finally being recognized, appreciated, and supported by government and non-
governmental agencies. In Mexico, as in countries around the world,
the spread of modern contraception coincided with feminist demands
that women's health issues, including, but not limited to, gynecological
matters, receive the attention they deserved, and be financed in con-
junction with new family planning promotions.

In government, foundation, and family planning agency documents
of the time, men were rarely mentioned as relevant to the new population programs. Perhaps they were overlooked by accident. Perhaps this
was an inadvertent consequence of women reasonably being made the
highest priority. Or perhaps there were underlying assumptions about
men, their biologies, and their essential interests and inclinations
when it came to sex and babies that precluded making them central to
campaigns around contraception, birth spacing, the optimal number
of children, and sexual health.

The not-so-invisible bias in the family planning room begs the
question: Are men reliable sexual partners, or are we better off leaving things to those who actually get pregnant? Weren't Mexican men
notorious machos? It was widely believed that for macho men, their
manhood and sense of self was intricately tied to proving their virility through procreation in general, through demonstrating degrees of
manliness through siring more offspring, and, to top it off, through
having as many male babies as possible. And weren't poor Mexican
men the worst of all? How to prevent the supposed inborn reluctance
by men to want to limit the number of children they had, and their
corresponding instinctive inability to be loving and respectful in sexual
relationships, from becoming impediments in the overall campaign to
disseminate information and contraception to women? Family planning across Mexico in the 1970s and 1980s could proceed even if men
were unenthusiastic about its goals and means—but if men were too
close-minded about birth control, for instance, they could become real
obstacles to achieving the main objectives of the program. Hence those

implementing the new policies around the country made it their aim
to provide contraceptives and information to women and make women
their sole focus of attention.

The personnel organizing reproductive health campaigns for women
at least implicitly assumed that Mexican men as a group, especially those
from the lower classes, were one-dimensional creatures who routinely
confounded the potency of their seed with their manly worth. There
were entire books about Mexican identity built around such characterizations of poor Mexican men, urban and rural, and they continued to be
read and taught throughout this period.

As in every other country on earth, in Mexico it was always possible to find examples from personal experience to prove these taken-
for-granted truths about irresponsible men. Fathers, brothers, husbands,
and sons who were especially brutish when it came to using protection,
sleeping around, and being a negligent father, at least when the children
were small, were common tropes. In the twentieth century, in Mexico
as in many other countries, canonical works defined the problems people suffered by focusing on poor men for a catalog of sins that held the
country back from becoming a cosmopolitan, modern society.[15]

There was a certain tautology in the argument. By omitting them
in policy documents, men seemed irrelevant when it came to family
planning. After all, women were clamoring for birth control. But where
were the men? At which point everyone could circle back and decry
men's lack of participation in family planning. So men were inadvertently written out of planning altogether.

Such marginalization by population specialists was premised on the
belief that men couldn't control themselves or be relied upon to behave in sexually respectable ways. If the government wanted to lower
birthrates, they would have to do so by concentrating their efforts rather
exclusively on women of reproductive age. In the first two decades of the
new century, these practices continued. The government health agencies went so far as to promote a program called the Oferta Sistemática
(Standard Offer): whenever a woman between fifteen and forty-nine

years old appeared at a government health clinic or hospital in need of assistance—recurring migraines or bronchitis or skin lesions or any other problem or symptoms—medical personnel were instructed to talk with her about birth control. Do you use something? Have you had any problems with your method? If you don't use contraception, why not? Unless a man accompanied a woman to the medical appointment, he was not party to such a line of inquiry, much less the focus of these questions.

It was not always this way. Did men do anything to prevent pregnancies before the advent of the birth control pill and the widespread availability of modern birth control for women? In Mexico men used condoms, and they practiced rhythm methods as best they could. They also achieved high marks from their wives on the manliness scale when they proved expert at the self-control required for withdrawal to work as a method of natural birth control. But it was only years after the fact that scholars seriously inquired about men's sexual practices in the past. It turned out that the widespread assumptions of previous years were incorrect: men in Mexico had demonstrated self-control, love, and a desire to space out children by learning when to pull out. Undoubtedly for some men this was a way of demonstrating that they had control over the situation, as though by withdrawing or not, a man could decide whether to try to avoid, risk, or try getting a woman pregnant. Withdrawal during sex was also, for some men, a way to share the burdens of planning when and how often to have children.[16]

All this was in the past. By the 1970s and later years, men, at best, became subjected to family planning's benign neglect. Unexamined conventions on the part of those responsible in government and private agencies about men and their sexuality had real consequences for promoting a gendered vision of responsibility for contraception.

WHAT WE DON'T KNOW HAS HURT US

When we think about men and sex, there may be a tendency to think the topic well covered and understood. Yet if we assumed less and risked more we might be surprised. Take a specific case of men and contraception—male sterilization, and who opts for this form of birth control and why. I studied vasectomies in the southern Mexican provincial capital of Oaxaca, and while this example might seem overly particular, unique even, we can draw lessons to shed light on the changing connections between men, sex, and their relationships with women more broadly.

Male sterilization in Mexico has never caught on in large numbers. In the early 2000s, the population in the state of Oaxaca was around 3.5 million. Approximately 3,000 of these inhabitants were men who had received vasectomies. This number was low by world standards, and the question I had was why so few Oaxacans had taken this route, and whether there were any sociodemographic patterns in the kind of men seeking sterilization. The explanation of public health personnel in Oaxaca was that men weren't interested or reliable when it came to birth control, and that men feared they would lose their potency if they received vasectomies. These conclusions helped account for why Mexican efforts to stem population growth continued to focus on the adoption of contraception for women, including tubal ligations.

The prevalence of vasectomy varies tremendously around the world, from a high in New Zealand of 19.3 percent of adult males (in 1995) to less than 2 percent in much of Africa and Latin America. China's rate was 6.7 percent in 2004; Iran's 2.8 percent in 2000; India's 1 percent in 2006, and in the United States the rate in 2002 was 12.8 percent. Mexico's rate overall was 1.9 percent in 2003, but the state of Oaxaca's was less than 1 percent. You might think that we would be able to predict different vasectomy rates based on different "national cultures," but you'd be wrong: the rate in the United Kingdom was around 18 percent in 1993, but then plummeted by 2016, when public funding for the procedure dried up.[17]

Even regions within the same country can vary widely. Take New Jersey and Idaho in 2002, for example: one of them had a vasectomy rate of 4.7 percent, and the other 19.9 percent. Guess which is which? Idaho's rate, 19.9 percent, was the highest rate in the country that year, and was followed numerically by Washington, Vermont, Oregon, Minnesota, Montana, New Hampshire, and Michigan (coming in at 15.7 percent). Something about those cold temperatures, no doubt, makes men more planful, or at least makes them want to have sex without worrying about pregnancies. What we don't know about men and sex. . . . [18]

In order to understand why men do or don't elect sterilization, we need to understand men's experiences, fears, desires, and relationships with women. I attended twenty-two vasectomies at clinics in Oaxaca City, talking with the patient up by his head as the surgeon did the snipping down below. You could say I provided emotional anesthesia for men undergoing the operation. It was usually a simple and quick procedure, but many men were nervous. I started by saying, "Well, they did this to me a few years ago," and let the conversation develop from there. Men would ask me in vague terms about my sexual performance after vasectomy. I would answer even more vaguely, but told them not to worry about a thing. Once a doctor asked me to take photographs of the event; I asked the patient, and to my surprise he agreed on the condition that I make copies of the photos and drop them off at the gas station where he worked. He wanted to share the moment with his family and friends.

I wanted to know whether there was a pattern in the kind of man seeking sterilization. I went in with the working assumption that the men would be drawn from the more educated, wealthier strata of Oaxaca society. I was quickly disabused of this notion. The men came from a wide range of backgrounds, and recommendations from friends and family, by word of mouth, proved a more significant factor in the decision than class or other social or cultural characteristics. [19]

The most telling commonality between men who got vasectomies revolved around the word "suffering." When I asked them why they had chosen to get sterilized, one man after another told me his wife had used contraception for decades, with time off birth control to get pregnant and give birth to two or three children. The women had suffered long enough; now it was their turn to share the burden. Men's relationships

with their wives or significant others, rather than schooling or employment type, lay behind more of the decisions to get a vasectomy than
any other factor. These men did not fit the stereotype in which men's
sexuality stands in stark contrast to women's. They shared a different perspective, defying all the theories of scholars about men needing to spread
their seed. With the women in their lives, they were intimately involved
in renegotiating the meanings of manhood and men's sexuality as well as
women's sexual and reproductive health.

Colombian anthropologist Mara Viveros has developed a concept
she calls "female contraceptive culture," in which women are the ones
responsible for preventing pregnancies. My friends in Oaxaca stand in
contrast to such notions, an unconditional refutation of the idea that
men cannot be trusted with so consequential a responsibility as helping
to decide whether and when a child should be brought into the world.[20]

It's tricky, of course, and getting a vasectomy means nothing in itself.
For some it is an act of love and generosity; for others it is an extension
of the most banal, hypermasculine traits. Getting a vasectomy involves
acting like a man, but what acting like a man exactly means can be
more difficult to discern. As we develop critiques that speak to social
inequalities, we invariably describe scenarios of who's to blame. When
we emphasize ideas about men being irresponsible around family planning, we can end up reinforcing relationships we want to change. When
we naturalize male sexuality, we say, to all intents and purposes, that
men have little choice in how they behave.

There was one gentlemen I encountered in the vasectomy clinics in
Oaxaca whose story seemed at first glance perverse. Before the surgery,
the nurse had a questionnaire to complete with Alejandro:

"Age?"

"40."

"Marital status?"

"Married."

"Children?"

"Two."

"Reason for having a vasectomy?"

"I don't want any more children."

"Previous birth control?"

Alejandro paused, finally answering, "None."

I followed up from my interview during Alejandro's operation to speak with him and his wife, Mercedes, a few days later in their home. I asked more about his reasons for getting a vasectomy. Mercedes answered instead of Alejandro:

"We'd been talking about it for eight years. Ever since our son was born."

Alejandro then clarified: "It was my idea. I decided to do it. I did it to satisfy her, not because I am going to sprinkle children around. Because she's already had her tubes tied, so . . . well . . . "

I was flummoxed. "If Mercedes has already done that, then why . . . ?"

"To please me," Mercedes said with tenderness.

"Why was this important to you?" I pressed her.

"Better to avoid surprises."

At which point Alejandro repeated his cheeky rejoinder: "So I don't go around sprinkling children everywhere. That's what she says."[21]

"Mexican men are like that, just like that," Mercedes said, ending the conversation.

Men's sexualized relationships with women are often overlooked in studies of men and masculinities. Taking the case of vasectomies, the postoperative "Will it work?" is not simply a question of erections and ejaculation. Men's anxieties about vasectomy and manhood are regularly linked in their minds to whether they will still be able to sexually satisfy a woman. With earnest sincerity, a man once commented that his favorite word to hear was "¡Así!" (Like that!). He never felt more like a man than when a woman in the heat of passion whispered to him, "Just like that!"

The meanings and consequences of men being "sexually uncontrollable" look different if we see men as "culture-bound," or as the housing-for-hormones out of control. Either way, these stereotypes complicate life for men who choose sterilization and want to challenge the stick-figure sexuality they have been assigned, as they must buck not just amorphous social constraints but also the actual ideas of family, friends, and medical personnel in the flesh about men and sex.

A final episode from the vasectomy chronicles sheds further light on efforts by government agents to force their judgments about men and sex on unsuspecting male populations: from 1975 to 1977, the prime minister of India, Indira Gandhi, launched mass sterilizations throughout India. In the end, 6.2 million more men and 2.1 million more women were left sterile after these two years. More men were sterilized because the procedure is easier and quicker to perform on men. In only one month, September 1976, health authorities carried out over 1.7 million sterilizations by sweeping into towns, rounding up all the males over the age of fifteen, dragging them to clinics, and forcibly sterilizing them. Among the main concerns of the men who were forcibly sterilized was that their vasectomies would rob them of virility and they would never again be able to sexually fulfill their wives.[22]

We can never understand the subject of men and sex unless we firmly grasp that for many heterosexual men their relationships with women deeply affect their motivations and actions. The definition of "manly" for these men is often "not womanly." For such men, their sense of worth as men is dependent in part on what they perceive to be women's assessment of their male attributes. Women's influence on male children has long been chronicled and analyzed by psychologists and anthropologists. The part that adult males play in the lives of women is also well documented and scrutinized. Surprisingly lacking in scholarly and popular literatures is the part that women play in defining and shaping men and masculinity.

In India and Mexico, as everywhere else, heterosexual men often base their sense of sexual self-worth on their ability to pleasure women. The history of contraception around the world shows the exclusion of men from major efforts to reduce fertility rates and improve women's health. The people creating and leading these family planning campaigns are without a doubt some of the most enlightened and progressive on earth in matters of sexuality, gender relations, and issues of inequality. They nonetheless have unintentionally been responsible for disseminating and highlighting some of our most parochial, pseudoscience attitudes and practices about men and sex.

A MIDWIFE'S CODA

After spending a year shadowing biomedical doctors in Oaxaca, I came to the inescapable conclusion that in their minds, men were sexually rapacious and women were sexual gatekeepers. The profligate male stood in full contrast to the persnickety female. For these doctors, the binary world of sexuality was invariably true not just in Oaxaca in the 2000s but also everywhere else in the world. That was just the nature of men's sexualities as compared to women's. Whenever I asked them about it, they responded that men want to have sex more than women do, and that they are more receptive to having sex with strangers than are women. "You're a man, Mateo," they confessed to me. "So you already know that."

At the same time, one summer I began to seek out another group of medical specialists, the indigenous healers and midwives who live throughout the mountainous state of Oaxaca. These practitioners call the hospital and clinic people "white-coat doctors," to tease them for their need to dress a certain way to impress their patients and set themselves sartorially apart from them. The indigenous healers and midwives weren't armed with years of formal medical training or bookcases of textbooks on morphology, anatomy, and physiology, but that didn't stop them from speaking knowledgably about the male afflictions of impotence, infertility, and infidelity.

Even though they practiced in villages and towns quite remote from one another, their responses when I asked about men's and women's sexual natures was remarkably similar. "Well, Mateo, that depends on the individual, doesn't it?" they might say. A static, dichotomous view of sexuality did not correspond to their conceptual framework; they had not witnessed this neat division in their medical practices. I wanted to know how they treated men's sexual problems. It was quickly apparent that not everyone in Oaxaca whose work involved thinking about men's and women's bodies and sexuality was as comfortable dividing the world into neat male/female categories. One midwife counseled, "It's important to get rid of the fear." She told me about a man she treated. "Now it turns out there were problems in his house. He saw his father do different things. My grandma used to tell me (when I was grown up, not when I was little), 'There are children who see their parents [have sexual relations]. It traumatizes them!' But why does it traumatize them? They want to know, 'How could our father use a woman like that?!'"[23]

These healers would no more generalize about men's sexualities than they would try to decipher some deep significance from the length of a woman's labor, and then compare how many hours different births took, to draw conclusions about the nature of the mothers. You could probably force a correlation, but at what cost to the poor mothers?

The harm in exaggerating the differences between men's and women's sexualities as inevitable, you could say, was not just that it was inaccurate, but that it led to favoring health treatments based on beliefs about men's and women's bodies that were not necessarily true. Biases are not valid reasons for pursuing health protocols. Nor is it appropriate to assume that certain thinking, desires, and behavior arise inevitably because someone is male or female.

Knowledge about men's sexuality does not necessarily run parallel with prevailing modern scientific ideas and practices, and men are not universally seen as sexually insatiable, or women deemed sexually hard to please, despite whatever we may have come to believe in recent years. Many of the ideas we assume to be true about men and women are historically specific beliefs camouflaged by scientific terms and pretense that have developed over the past one hundred or so years. Renewed attention to women's libido often describes it as "more like men's than we realized." That women's sexuality is not inherently passive is a revelation. That women's sexual pleasure was denied in scientific literature for most of the twentieth century is a real problem. That we still repeat trite notions about men's sexual pleasure is also a problem.

There is good news, however. As Rebecca Jordan-Young reported in her 2010 book *Brain Storm*, "high libido, multiple partners, and more varied and frequent sexual activities are all treated as part of normal female sexuality in more recent brain organization studies, even though each of these was previously interpreted as a masculine sexual pattern." That neuroscientists' findings coincide with changing social attitudes and practices when it comes to women and sexuality seems more than a coincidence.[24]

What we think about men and sex—are we normal or anomalous?— may have less to do with our own experiences and more to do with whom we listen to about our experiences. This is equally true of that other lightning-rod issue regarding men's biological penchants: violence. The connections between men, sex, and violence are never in sharper relief than when it comes to understanding rape, that insidious violence that deploys sex to wreak its damage.

CHAPTER FIVE

MEN'S NATURAL AGGRESSIONS

It is . . . in risking life that man is raised above the animal;
that is why superiority has been accorded in humanity
not to the sex that brings forth but to that which kills.

SIMONE DE BEAUVOIR

M EN CAUSE WAR.

Aristophanes knew how to stop men's wars when he wrote *Lysistrata*: women should deny men sex. Spike Lee knew how when he filmed *Chi-Raq*: women should deny men sex. Susan Sontag, channeling Virginia Woolf, taunted that war is a man's game, and the killing machine has a gender: it is male. She seemed to believe not only that men make war but that (most) men like war. How long has that truism tyrannized martial thought?[1]

From domestic abuse to international terrorism, the common denominator in contemporary discussions of violence is men. For several decades, cultural anthropologists have studied and analyzed masculinities and gender-based violence of all sorts. Meanwhile, biological anthropologists have examined how evolutionary processes, genomics, and endocrinology relate to maleness and violence. We are all trying to untangle the manly roots of violence.

Certain ideas about men, aggression, violence, and war are so wide-spread that when a credentialed author comes along who confirms what people think they already know—that men are habitually inclined to fight for what they want—we find ourselves in a kind of feedback loop of misinformation. Men are more violent than women, right? They have murdered and raped in far higher numbers throughout history in every known culture on earth. Plenty of studies extrapolate from male chimpanzees to humans to argue that sexually aggressive males have more offspring, thus supposedly fulfilling their evolutionary promise. This analogy is a harmful overstatement making rape seem more natural in the animal kingdom than it is and implying that all men have an enduring biological potential to commit rape.

In order to understand aggression in males of the human species, we need to step back and ask, first of all, if it really makes sense to say men are more violent than women, and, second, whether patterns of male aggression and violence really are universal. To repeat an earlier point, it is not the same thing to say "men murder" as it is to say "most murderers are men." Most men don't murder or rape or engage in violent behavior. Studies of aggressive behavior in couple relationships in the United States in fact point to similar rates for women and men of screaming and other forms of verbal abuse, slamming doors, slapping, pushing, throwing things, and hitting. The more extreme, dangerous, harmful, and deadly types of domestic violence are perpetrated more often by men than women. The milder forms of violence are most frequently seen with young couples, especially while they are dating.[2]

And it's not just a matter of strength. It is no more helpful to say that the reason men beat women more than women beat men is because they are naturally stronger than it is to say that mothers beat their children more than children beat their mothers because the mothers are stronger. Control, power, protection, and authority are the keys to understanding violence and aggression; they are culturally and not simply biologically embedded.

Crucially, societies in which women have more power usually have a lower incidence of male-on-female violence and aggression than societies in which they have less power. Relationships between men and between women also make a difference: specifically, as biopsychologist Barbara Smuts wrote in a famous 1992 paper on cross-cultural variation and male aggression, "the form and frequency of male violence against women is related to the nature of men's relationships with one another," and "the nature of female relationships influences female vulnerability to male aggression."[3]

Claims that women are less naturally aggressive than men have been used to keep women from combat assignments in militaries throughout history. Not infrequently, certain populations of men—poor men, Wall Street men, African men, Mexican men, urban men, rural men—are tagged as especially prone to violence, little able to control primordial male urges to act out hostilities. The jargon that accompanies these arguments lends them an air of objectivity, using terms such as "selfish genes," "demonic males," "the spread of agriculture," "psychopathology," and "politics by other means." Yet as soon as we hear that there are more or less violent men, or about variations in rates of male violence from one group to another, or one historical period to another, we should begin to suspect a fatal defect in the reasoning. Extreme versions of biological explanations of male violence get us nowhere. We still need to explore why violence is perpetrated by men more than women, and we need to understand the pervasiveness of rape and the perniciousness of rape culture. But we should now be able to avoid casual language like "men are more violent than women." Men as a physiological category are not violent. Some men are violent some of the time. Men as a uniform category do not rape. Some men do some of the time. If we want to stop these men we need to make sure we understand why.[4]

All this still begs the question of why violence has been perpetrated by men more often than by women around the world and throughout history. The first point to make, again, is that it depends what you call violence, because women commit some forms of violence as much as men. A key distinction is lethality, with far more men than women involved in life-threatening forms of violence today and historically. If the reason men murder and rape and are killed in far higher numbers than women is not about biology, then what are the social factors driving these deadly forms of violence? The answer is as simple and complicated as the patriarchy and dwells in the broader nature of male privilege at the level of states, corporations, and other social institutions as well as in more intimate settings, from communities to families.

Violence is employed to impose control over others, whether it's about one family or individual against another or one country, class, or racial group against another. To the extent that men dominate the entities involved—whether states or families—the purpose of their violence is expressly to dictate their terms to others. The causes of individual, social, and political violence cannot be condensed simplistically to patriarchal systems of rule, but it would be hard not to connect masculinity to militarism and domestic violence. So there certainly appears to be something distinctive in contemporary societies connecting men, maleness, and masculinity with violence and aggression. It's important we excise prevalent but erroneous beliefs about what is chronic and what is situational about manly belligerence.

SELECTIVE MUSTERING

I sometimes ask students in my undergraduate classes how many of them who are US citizens reported to a government agency when they turned eighteen. Usually about half the American students raise their hands. Why half? Because only young men in the United States are required to register with the US Selective Service System (SSS) on that birthday to ensure that all eligible young men are enrolled in the event of a future military draft.

Why only young men? This answer is not so easy. Depending on how you count, there are around seventy countries in the world that practice some form of conscription. With few exceptions, only young men are conscripted into the armed forces of their respective countries, and in these countries, military service is compulsory only for males of a certain age. Even in countries without conscription, of course, the armed forces make close associations between men, masculinity, sacrifice, and service.[5]

The notion of "service" is itself highly charged: to serve in a citizen army is often regarded as the most heightened form of modern male experience, an almost sacred duty. Those who engage in this form of sacrifice for the national good are prototypically male. Even when lives are not at stake, military training promises to teach young men skills and trades that will be crucial as they prepare for their consummate male breadwinner duties. Together with voting, joining the military in the United States is touted as the embodiment of democratic citizenship. Deployment promises youths, especially poor and male youths, with practical rewards, in the form of jobs, as well as idealized incentives, such as honor. Enlistment is presented to recruits not only as a way to serve the country and contribute to the broader good of society, but as a path to personal growth and a way out of poverty. This is as true for female recruits, who make up 15 percent of the enlisted ranks in the United States, as it is for male recruits.

The justifications in the 2010s for drafting only young men, and for the fact that 85 percent of the US armed forces is male, are historical, comparative, and physical, going back to the days when warriors were expected to carry shields and swords into battle. Since time immemorial, men have fought wars everywhere in the world. Perhaps we might explain male-only conscription through some form of collective unconscious, and our memories of who carried the spears, and later the crossbows, have led us to male-only conscription today. Even if that's not the case, cultural considerations—such as core convictions about male and female aptitudes, emotions, and predispositions, substantiated by ideas about biological differences—certainly play an important role in military recruitment practices and policies.

As of 2014, 22 million people in the United States were military veterans, and 16.5 million of these were classified as "wartime vets" (from World War II, Korea, Vietnam, Iraq, and Afghanistan). That means about 7 percent of the population, or one in every fourteen people (1.3 percent of women and 13.4 percent of men), had been in the military at some point in their lives. It also means that in 2014, almost one out of every seven adult men in the United States was a veteran. These numbers help shape thinking around men and the military and reveal the sway of the warrior mentality throughout US society. As the largest employer in the country, the US armed forces are also dominant players in directing US relations with the rest of the world, with more troops stationed outside the borders of the nation than the military forces of any other country in history.

The US military has always reflected general patterns of class and regional divisions in the country. In the opening decades of the twenty-first century, young men, and to a lesser extent young women, without economic, political, or cultural clout continued to be recruited to carry out the United States' requirements of invasion, occupation, and post-conflict pacification. They were drawn disproportionately from certain regions, such as the southeastern United States. Since the rise of citizen armies and the revolutionary French *levée en masse*, the most marginal sectors of society have been lured into the military's lowest rungs. It has not necessarily been a question of tricking young men into enlistment; young men have always found plenty of reasons to join the military, train, and embrace deployment, even in war zones.

The history of conscription in the United States is a history of press-ganging and seducing young men into uniform to risk life and limb, to kill and be killed. Registration was sometimes mandatory, but sometimes not. The draft that had been in place for most of the twentieth century officially ended in July 1973, when the so-called All-Volunteer Force (AVF) began operating. Between 1975 and 1980, registration was voluntary.

In 1980, after the Soviet Union invaded Afghanistan, President Jimmy Carter reinstated registration for eighteen-year-old men. Since that time, the US government has required all men to register for the draft when they turn eighteen. Although women accounted for only 1.1 percent of active-duty personnel in 1970, the Pentagon began recruiting the hell out of women in the late 1970s. Women accounted for 8.5 percent of enlisted forces by 1980 and around 15 percent by 2000.[6]

Historically military service has offered a way for the most dispossessed members of American society to achieve the pinnacle of democratic citizenship. Yet the bromide of democracy in which citizens, especially male youths, will take up arms if and when requested by the nation-state is losing whatever formulaic allure it may have once held for millions of young men. The War on Terrorism declared by the US government seems as endless as it is senseless, but to conduct this war the government must not only retain public support for its efforts in general but more specifically continue to motivate millions of its young men to serve in the military and wage war.

TINA'S KNIFE AND DEMOND'S LAST MISSION

Tina Garnanez is an Iraq War veteran. I met her in late 2005, not long after she returned from the front. She had been a medic there and nicknamed her ambulance partner Newt. They masqueraded as husband and wife, even wearing wedding rings, to keep the men at bay when they tried to hit on Tina. Newt made sure no one messed with her.

"He's a big, big boy. I liked that. He took care of me. He spoiled me rotten and I loved it," Tina told me. "He got me food and always kept me warm. He made me feel very safe." If someone started to harass her, she'd look around, find Newt, and shout out, "Where's my husband? *There's* my husband!" And Newt would come over.

But there were some problems Newt couldn't solve for Tina. Like missing her girlfriend. "I was in a relationship back home when I was in

Iraq, and it helped me, God it helped me. It was my sanity, you know?" Other soldiers would sometimes ask, "Why do you have a picture of a girl on your wall?" She put up other photos to confuse everybody. Men had to be told no fifty times before they got the message. She wanted to tell them, "You're barking up the wrong tree."

In Iraq and generally in the military, Tina found, "Women were often seen as either promiscuous or lesbians. I just didn't think it was fair that I had to pretend to be straight." Meanwhile, she had signed up for only four years in the army but then got "stop-lossed," held over for another tour of Iraq. Mosul, Balad, Kirkuk. Convoys. IEDs. Wounded. One-hour catnaps. Meals-Ready-to-Eat. Sand. Heat. But that was never the worst of it. "It's very sad, just being a woman out there," she said. On one base, the Morale, Welfare, and Recreation shack was a good half-mile from where Tina slept. If she wanted to check her email or call home, she had to go there. If she got back from a convoy at two in the morning, well, that might be the best time to call her mom in New Mexico.

"I would call her and then I'd have to walk all the way back in the dark. I was always ready with my knife. I'd sort of have it open, have it tucked away a little. Just ready, so I could pull it out. I was listening constantly. The road was gravel and so I'd walk in the grass next to the road, and if someone was behind me, I could hear them on the gravel."

Tina grew quiet as she recounted more of her story to me. She'd come back to the Southwest, to reconnect with her family, with her Navajo ways, and with the arid countryside, where she could sometimes get away from the bustle of people. The consequences of encountering and avoiding men who could bring violence on Tina forced her to think about lifelong experiences of abuse at the hands of men. It helped her develop a defensive stance to cope with every new threat that could come her way.

"I was so angry at the fact that not only did I have to worry about dying on these convoys, but I'd worry about coming back to the base, about my fellow soldiers doing something to me. That really, really bothered me," she said. She told me that before she was in the military, she had been abused. "So I've always had an attitude of, 'Hey, men are dangerous.' I don't really trust men too much. And then to be in the military and have all the unwanted advances by older men. That just rubbed me the wrong way and scared me."

But the associations between men and violence in the military do not impact just women. In Demond Mullins's case, the connection was different but also disconcerting. In Demond's last days and hours in Iraq, he began to realize that the worst was over. He was going to make it home in one piece. He had taken nothing for granted. But he would not be among those who returned home with grotesque burns and mangled or missing limbs; he would not be facing dozens of surgeries and months and years of painful rehab.[7]

"When I came in from my last mission in Iraq," he told me several years later, "as we drove into the camp there were all these people from my company to greet us. And we were all shouting, 'Wow, this is our last mission! We made it! We're going home alive!' My executive officer [XO] walked up to me and said, 'You're a man now!' That's what he said to me. And I thought about that, and I still think about that now. Is it violence, is it acts of violence that make me a man? Or is it my potential for violence that make me manly or masculine?" For Demond, the consequences of *being* a man of violence, a man who had witnessed violence and had committed violence, meant that he had to come to grips with whether the violence he'd brought down on the Iraqis had always lain dormant, latent inside him, waiting to be unleashed by war, or was something alien that had been rammed into him by military circumstance.

The comment that after participating in violence in Iraq he was now a man did not sit well with Demond: "I think that the military really plays on that," he said. "From childhood, you're socialized into your ideology of what masculinity is or what manhood is. And pop culture plays on that well. When you're too young to get into the military, you're fed these images. Then, just joining the military, it's like you're trying to prove that you are a man. And to say you're a man because 'I experienced combat.' Well, how did that make me a man?"[8]

The XO's congratulations were not so much a cultural slap on the back—"You learned through your experiences how to be a man"—as an acknowledgment that war was what allowed Demond to activate his inner warrior. It had been there all along, sitting inactive, and just required the right conditions to be unleashed through the crucible of war. The XO would never have exclaimed to a woman soldier, "You're a woman now!"

Demond continued, "I was twenty-two when I first went to Iraq. I was already a man. Do my violent acts make me an alpha male among civilians now? It's messed up, because even though I know all this, I internalized what I learned." He found escape from the pain and suicidal feelings through what he called "nihility," which "makes me feel comfortable. I'm like, 'You don't have a pot to piss in. Everybody's in pretty bad shape because we're all just trying to make it. Some people are really well off, and some people are not.' This actually comforts me. There's some people that it scares, that life has no point, no structure. To me, I'm comforted by it."

Nothingness and distrust had captured Demond's manly warrior spirit. As an African American man he was used to people telling him their opinions about masculinity and aggression and what makes a good team player. In the disjuncture between societal bromides about men and war and the maw of actual war in Iraq, Demond returned home with a quiet resolve to disprove each and every one of those patently militaristic banalities about war releasing his inner manhood.

WHY MEN MAKE WAR

Anyone from the United States who has spent much time abroad has been faced with the question, "Why are you Americans so violent? So many mass murders. So many wars." But it's not just Americans who are associated with violence and war making; militarism exists in every land, and it always has a male face. Except in science fiction and Greek mythology, there have never been armies of women who singlehandedly invaded, occupied, and subjugated enemy populations.

The associations between men, maleness, violence, and warfare are ubiquitous, and that can easily lead to the belief that there is something natural to men and aggressiveness, making it all the more important to unpack naturalist arguments about the causes of war and men's violent tendencies. How gendered these qualities are seen to be has immediate significance for our overmilitarized societies. In the late twentieth and early twenty-first centuries, a new spate of learned reports on the origins of war revived a simple set of explanations.

One version of the naturalist argument about men and aggression that continues to hold traction is the hormonal hypothesis. In the words of Cambridge neuroscientist Joe Herbert, writing in 2015, "the occurrence of war may simply be an inevitable result of the powerful effects that testosterone has on male motivation, competitiveness, ambition, and risk-taking." Furthermore, "testosterone is thus an essential contributor to the emergence of the war-like male responsible for the phenomenon of war." Whether generals are supposed to have higher levels of testosterone than other people to begin with, or their levels are thought to rise after they start issuing commands to attack, the hormonal hypothesis makes the origins of war one of chemical reaction. So much for gold, slaves, oil, and territory.[9]

Another notable naturalist argument linking men and war concerns paternity, or rather, what is known in the trade as "paternity uncertainty." The argument is a who-knows-whom-I've-sired for the Age of DNA, and it has both clarified and muddied the significance of bloodlines and, it turns out, the origins of war.

My friend Richard Bribiescas teaches biological anthropology at Yale. I always learn a lot from my discussions with him about evolution and hormones in men. That doesn't mean we always see eye to eye. Writing in *Men: Evolutionary and Life History*, Bribiescas asks, "So why is it that women tend to invest more time and energy in offspring than men do?" The answer, he says, "lies in the simple factor of parental identification." Whereas others have argued that the accident of evolution entrusting pregnancy and lactation to women is the best way to explain divisions of labor between parents going back tens of thousands of years, Bribiescas underscores another consequence of evolutionary theory: the presumed universal misgivings men have about their ability to corroborate the harvest of their seed.

"The questions facing males are: Are my children really mine?" Bribiescas asks. This leads him to a big theme of his book: "the central role of paternity uncertainty in human male evolution." Women, Bribiescas says, "are the only people who can assuredly identify those who are genetically related to them. Men can never have the same assurance. From an evolutionary perspective, males are quite alone." In addition, and crucially, because of their solitary condition, because men don't know who their offspring are, they feel less reticence about going to war. Men invest less in child-rearing, and because of this lack of allegiance to others they have supposedly been more prone to wage war historically. In essence, they have not cared about whom they might kill.

Here is the logic: "Without the inhibitions that result from not wanting to harm their offspring or their kin, men might well be less restrained than women in their actions, at a personal and global level." Bribiescas is worried (as any thinking person should be) about the old men whose fingers are on the actual buttons of nuclear war. In case the full implications of this thesis are still not clear, he concludes: "Men wage war because they can and because the potential costs of such action to their evolutionary fitness may be zero."[10]

When I interviewed him in 2015 in New Haven, Connecticut, Bribiescas could not have been more receptive when I raised my concerns. With no other species is the threat of thermonuclear annihilation so present when males make war, I noted, and therefore, with no other species do the causes of war matter so much. Yes, he agreed, and he admitted that it made little sense to propose paternity uncertainty as the proximate cause in a general's mind when he sends men into combat. In part, he meant these speculative thoughts as a provocation to further discussion about men and war. (As he likes to say: "An idea is like a cockroach. Put it on the table, and if you can't kill it, well, then maybe it's meant to survive.") I admitted to being provoked: Why does not knowing who your offspring are make men more cavalier about whom they kill in battle, as opposed to being more reluctant to go to war and kill possible progeny? The question, for scientist and layperson alike, is at what cost do we consider reasonable the hypothesis that "men wage war because they can and because the potential costs of such action to their evolutionary fitness may be zero"?

Without assuming that the assassin of Archduke Ferdinand or the kamikaze pilots over Pearl Harbor had fatherhood issues that caused them to go off to war, where this leaves the rumble of empire, the economics of slavery, and the surge of national liberation movements is unclear except that in each case there is an underlying logic of fatherly ignorance. Could Bribiescas be right that, at least from an evolutionary perspective, fatherly ignorance is a constant and key catalyst to warfare? That conclusion is consistent with certain prevalent versions of evolutionary theory, beginning with war as the outcome of primordial doubts and decision making. Despite the fact that in most societies around the world, today and historically, women rely for security on men who are not in any way genetically related to them, theories that connect men and evolution to war can easily resonate with a wide public.

Obviously, then, if all it would take to stop war, end bloated military budgets, and cease all the interventions are paternity tests, we could quickly convince the men who roam the earth with their reckless germ to knock it off. The point that my friend was making was nothing so simplistic, but his argument could reinforce the idea that the origins of war have more to do with evolution and male biology than is the case. To explain why we take easy comfort in paternity uncertainty as an explanation for war, we might consider the power of wishes, and how the wish to understand can trump the wish for things to be otherwise. If we can explain in an elemental way that war results from the ambiguous nature of paternity, and if we are pretty sure that males will continue to sire progeny, then at least we can know some of the limits on our ability to limit war and better avoid the fool's errand of contesting the evolutionary roots of war.

The predicament this line of thinking poses also relates to the difference between an error and an illusion. In discussing the resilience of religion, political philosopher Wendy Brown asks why religion does not collapse under the weight of illogic alone. The reason, she says, paraphrasing Freud, is that religion "is not merely an error, but an illusion." Brown clarifies: "Errors are mistakes, while an illusion is powered by a wish." Today wars continue despite mistaken goals and strategies, their existential error, you could say. And, as with religion, illusion is central to maintaining every war. Hypothesizing that war is caused by evolutionary controls and compulsions of paternity uncertainty could be called an error, but that would not explain the currency given to this error or others tracing the origins of war to the biologies of our male ancestors.[11]

Explanations for war may be illusory, yet war is far from an illusion. Moving people from illusions about war to engaging in the practices of war requires a conjurer's trick of symbolic reasoning and the ability to move people from one state of understanding to another. We need to better understand what maleness has to do with norms and categories—civilian, enlisted, tooth-to-tail, obedient, resourceful, intimidating and intimidated, weapons savvy and pacifistic—for the fog of war to be transcended and military conflict buried in the annals of history.

Man does not cause war. Particular men do, and the reason is always to impose their will on an opposing force.

SEA AMONG THE UN PEACEKEEPERS

The United Nations' peacekeeping forces have a significant problem of Sexual Exploitation and Abuse (SEA, pronounced S-E-A). Despite a zero-tolerance policy on missions around the world that prohibits sexual relations between UN personnel and members of the local population, almost no one in the United Nations believes this policy is feasible. Why they don't is directly relevant to widespread assumptions about men, war, and sexual violence. Blue Helmets have been caught buying sex, including from children, for a dollar, for eggs, for a cup of milk, for a cookie. In UN camps and cars, in towns and in the forest, in hotels, apartments, and everywhere else, women and girls as well as boys are targets for SEA. And peacekeeping soldiers and police are not the only ones who leave behind "Blue Helmet children" and "peacekeeper babies." UN civilian personnel are perhaps the biggest offenders. But regardless of a perpetrator's position, the United Nations would in most cases sooner repatriate an employee from a mission than arrest, prosecute, and punish him onsite.

A 2013 UN investigation into SEA concluded that "virtually all personnel knew about UN policies surrounding SEA," and that "the great majority of personnel do get trained." More and better training proved no more effective than "no-go areas," or making UN military and police wear uniforms with name tags, or hotlines for local women to use to report violations. Exercise equipment in barracks was imported to provide temporary and partial release of pent-up sexual energy among the troops.[12]

Assessments were issued beginning with the landmark 2005 "Comprehensive Strategy" report by Prince Zeid Ra'ad Al Hussein of Jordan, who at the time was adviser to the secretary-general on sexual exploitation and abuse. The report condemned such abuses and called for dramatically new procedures to eradicate the problem on UN peacekeeping missions around the world. Yet a culture of impunity continued to prevail. A primary cause of SEA proved to be underlying beliefs about male biology among UN officials, a boys-will-be-boys mentality with regard to men's elemental need for sexual release, even if this means violently exploiting women, girls, and boys, members of the very populations the peacekeepers were charged with protecting. The proposed solutions to the problem gleaned from interviews in Haiti and Lebanon fell into two categories: the first involving tours of duty and the hydraulic model, the second involving leaves and the safety-valve theory.[13]

As in all militarily volatile situations, in Haiti and Lebanon the length of time that soldiers and police were assigned to a UN mission was regulated and monitored. Commanding officers spoke in particular of the challenges for young male soldiers in their twenties being away from home in a foreign country for the first time. Some also drew a direct connection between length of tour and sexual exploitation. In the words of Daniel Morales, a police commander from Chile, "If you put men in a situation where they are not going to have sex for three months, that is a challenge, but not insurmountable. If you extend this to six months, well, that is far more difficult. Beyond this point they become unmanageable."[14]

One solution in the Chilean and Peruvian contingents was to make it possible for men to call home, including through Skype, nearly every day. The hope was less that the men's suppressed sexual drive would be relieved by talking to their wives and girlfriends back home than that talking to family would intensify guilty feelings if the men were tempted to have sex with local women. Peacekeeper men had their sexual needs, the logic ran; they could not be expected to endure celibacy forever. The longer the men were prevented from finding release for their sexual needs, the more the pressure would keep building. It was only reflexes at play when the men at some point sought an outlet before they exploded from sexual privation and denial of their sexual selves.

In Haiti, peacekeepers on leave were sent to the Dominican Republic because on the same island there were sex workers. What happened in the DR stayed in the DR and was not of interest to UN peacekeeping officials, much less considered to be their legal responsibility. In Lebanon, peacekeepers were shipped off for R&R to another country, such as Cyprus. The goal was simply to get them out of the southern zone in Lebanon where the UN contingents were based. In that case, what happened with peacekeepers on leave in Cyprus stayed in Cyprus. The Dominican Republic and Cyprus each played the role of safety valve for the UN peacekeepers. If and when the United Nations' male troops couldn't take the sexual stress any longer, they had somewhere to let off "steam" where it would not as directly affect the UN missions.

Concerns about men's biology directly influenced military tour and leave policies. Warrior masculinities have always been at the core of sexual exploitation and abuse in the UN peacekeeping forces and cannot be simply trained out or cordoned off. A code of physical endurance and conquest is at the heart of warrior masculinities, and carries with it the ethos of male privilege and prerogative that warriors deserve the spoils of war, which regularly include the bodies of civilian women. But it's more than a problem of armed men abusing their power. There is good evidence that more civilians than soldiers or police are responsible for SEA in many missions where the problem has been documented. This evidence implies something far more sinister than what happens to young men when they are given guns and unleashed in foreign lands. It was not warrior masculinities that were causing sexual exploitation and abuse, but any kind of masculinity—and for civilian personnel, the greater freedom and impunity they enjoyed: in Haiti, at least, civilians were allowed far more latitude in terms of mobility and supervision than peacekeeper soldiers and police.

These UN civilian employees do not generally carry weapons, so the abuse was not simply a matter of armed intimidation. Civilian personnel were, on average, older than the soldiers, so it was also not just a question of young men and their hormones. Masculine privilege and male entitlement among the peacekeepers, bolstered by commonsense beliefs about men's sexual needs, explain the problem far better than theories about soldiers who go bad or simply mothers who are so desperate for funds that they offer their daughters' bodies for sale.

RAPE AS NORMAL MALE SEXUALITY

"Suppose rape is rooted in a feature of human nature," writes psychologist Steven Pinker, "such as that men want sex across a wider range of circumstances than women do. It is *also* a feature of human nature, just as deeply rooted in our evolution, that women want control over when and with whom they have sex." Just because it's a feature of human nature, Pinker cautions, doesn't make it right. But it does make it natural in an evolutionary sense. Belittling environmentalists and others who idealize nature—people who believe "that anything we have inherited from this Eden is healthy and proper"—Pinker also criticizes the lack of sophistication of anyone who thinks "a claim that aggression or rape is 'natural,' in the sense of having been favored by evolution, is tantamount to saying that it is good." Isn't the world full of natural, beautiful, and necessary predators, such as wolves, bears, and sharks?[15]

For evolutionary psychologists and the behavioral geneticists who are their allies, rape is the touchstone case they use to promote the idea that key aspects of gender and sexuality are just too hardwired to ignore. Unless you understand the brutal, biological roots of male violence that takes the form of rape, which is found in all human societies and in species spread across the animal kingdom, they declare, you cannot effectively prevent rape. Everyone would agree that unless you understand the causes of rape you cannot stop it, and that if you get the causes wrong you will not only not solve the problem but make it worse. Rarely does scholarship matter more for public policy.[16]

"Nowhere else in modern intellectual life is the denial of human nature more passionately insisted upon, and nowhere else is the alternative more deeply misunderstood," writes Pinker. He adds, "Clarifying these issues, I believe, would go a long way toward reconciling three ideals that have needlessly been put into conflict: women's rights, a biologically informed understanding of human nature, and common sense." Especially, he might have added, if you're concerned about women's rights, you need to pay attention to the biological influences, drives, controls, and restrictions that govern who rapes whom, why, and when. Yet to call rape a feature of human nature makes no more sense than to say that opposing rape is a feature of human nature—it tells us nothing in itself, but it uncritically implies that something dangerous is permanently lodged in "male nature" that can harm others. Anthropologist Emily Martin's succinct response to the major study that inspired Pinker is apropos: "Protestations to the contrary, their account actually amounts to an incitement to rape."[17]

Pinker may be able to find rape in every society and historical period. But the tremendous variation of rates of rape is not a factor of biology. Why in 2014 were rates of reported rape in Alaska 79.7 for every 100,000 people, while in New Jersey the rate that same year was 11.7, according to FBI crime statistics? Presumably the biology of Alaskan males does not differ markedly from that of the men of New Jersey. When he does compare societies, Pinker suggests that greater freedom for women and independence from men could be spelling the threat of *more* danger, including with rape. "The targeting of sexist attitudes does not seem to be a particularly promising avenue for reducing rape," he says, yet his broad claims are not backed by evidence, as would be required to use his framework to explain that women of Alaska are 6.8 times as independent as women in New Jersey.[18]

The same variation that is found in the United States is also found when comparing rape in countries and regions across the globe as well as throughout history. Anthropologist Peggy Sanday writes about rape cross-culturally that, "To say that at least some men rape in all societies and to use this fact to make generalizations about the natural history of rape and the biological bases for sexual coercion obfuscates the dramatic cultural differences between a rape-free society . . . and a rape-prone society." A prime example of the latter, she believes, is the United States. Such variation leads to a question: If rape is so natural to the males of our species, why is it far less prevalent in some places than in others, and why does the incidence of rape instead correlate so closely with other social markers, such as gender equality?[19]

"Rape represents the breakdown of the normal social controls on male sexuality," reports neuroscientist Joe Herbert. Social controls in this scenario are all that can stop rape, and undoubtedly most of the people who lay rape at the feet of nature are pessimistic about ridding

rape from human societies altogether. As historian Joanna Bourke persuasively shows, if we try to trace rape back to universal biological roots,
this will result not only in public policies designed to control, cordon,
and quarantine men, but also the decision to literally castrate them.
Indeed, chemical and surgical castration is advocated and practiced, including in the United States, as a strategy to prevent rape. If the penis is
out of control, the reasoning goes, then the male genitals must be punished. "Invasive procedures like sterilization, castration and lobotomy
assumed that rape arose primarily as a result of uncontrollable sexual
urges" on the part of men, Bourke notes.[20]

Leaving aside Pinker's intemperate views—"Rapists tend to be los-
ers and nobodies," he says, "while presumably the main beneficiaries of
the patriarchy are the rich and powerful"—debate about rape and normal men has run the gamut for decades among feminists and activists.
Some have held that all men are basically beneficiaries of rape, while
others have gone so far as to call all men potential rapists. Both the
all-men-as-beneficiaries and the all-men-as-potential-rapists arguments
mingle too easily with notions of biological destiny. The Alaska–New
Jersey rape rate comparison is pertinent: instead of looking to biology,
or to the claim that rapists are poor, uneducated men who can't find another way to have sex, we need to grasp that rape is caused by inequality
and by the desire and ability of people, nearly always male, to sexually
impose their violent power and will over others.[21]

Men's bodies are no more in thrall to disobedient impulses than
women's. Men's bodies are no more in need of collective disciplining
than women's. Men's bodies are biologically no more or less choosy, coy,
or capricious than women's. Rape is not explained best by who gets erections. Men are not more enslaved by some rapacious nature, although
if you listened to some theorists, expert and non-expert alike, you might
believe they are. Men rape young women, men rape old women, men
rape children, men rape men, men rape in peacetime, men rape in
wartime, men rape in cities, men rape in rural areas. Although there
are blatant and pervasive patterns—rapists are men—it is possible not

to leap into believing it all has something to do with inherent maleness and male bodies.

If rape is biologically driven, and men can't help themselves, then who can stop them? Perhaps we could agree that "society must act against men's sexual assaults against women." But to say society must act is to say little, to depersonalize responsibility. Who is this "society"? If you think men can't help themselves, the single logical conclusion is that only women can stop men. And, following from this, if women don't stop men, they are in part responsible for what happens and can be blamed for not preventing rape. Of course, if they are thought to be helpless in the face of male sexual assault, women can only hope to be rescued by other men who don't assault. As Laura Kipnis writes, "policies and codes that bolster traditional femininity—which has always favored stories about female endangerment over stories about female agency—are the *last* thing in the world that's going to reduce sexual assault." Either way, men as a group are implicated in rape overall and men who rape are let off the hook.[22]

In order for rape to be considered natural, it must be true of all men, or human males, as the evolutionary psychologists like to call them, in all times and places. Variation spells problems. But not always. Because it turns out, according to the rape-is-natural folks, that "males of a lower socioeconomic status are more likely to rape." We've heard this before. This particular version is explained in a simple fashion: poorer men have a harder time getting anyone to have sex with them, and to compensate, because they have to follow their natural male sexual urges and find something to ejaculate into, they rape. If women are available, they are most often raped. If not, as in prison, then other men are raped. It all boils down to a "mate-deprivation hypothesis."[23]

To call something like rape by men natural and genetic (hidden in the barely controllable XY chromosomal combination) means that you cannot really stop rape at its source. You can only try to limit the damage male rapists can do to the rest of the population. Look again at variation: human males do or don't rape (to the extent we know it), and they do

or don't think about rape, and do or don't want to rape (same qualifi-
cation). If the range of thinking and doing among men is infinite, if we
can tell little to nothing about whether a man will rape simply because
we know he is a human male, then nature is surely taking a back seat to
other factors. Here we have another reason why it is beyond the pale to
label as rape what males of other species, like mallard ducks, do in a far
less flexible manner, in attacks that are almost identical in nature, carried out by a significant number of the species population, and appear
to be nearly unvarying.[24]

WHAT'S NATURAL AND GOOD

The only good thing to come out of rape culture in the United States
has been news coverage exposing it: the sexual assaults of entitled
men—from boardrooms to elite college dormitories—make it clear that
men of wealth and power can exploit male privilege just as much as
men from every other social sector. It's also reassuring that the problem
has come to be called rape *culture*, because that name helps to guard
against a presumption that rape is natural to the males of the human
and other species. But even when we read about rape culture, we need
to be wary of some of the underlying assumptions that can be reinforced
about the naturalness of rape, and how more men would if they could.

Do you remember this news item in one or another incarnation
from 2015?

"Nearly one-third of college men admit they might rape a woman
if they could get away with it, a new study on campus sexual assaults
claims. Of those men, however, far fewer will admit this if the word
rape is actually used during the course of questioning."

"Close to 1-in-3 collegiate males admitted in a recent study they
would force a woman to sexual intercourse, but many would not consider that rape."

"According to one study of male students at the University of North
Dakota, 1 in 3 men would rape a woman if they could get away with it."

"Nearly a third of college men in the US admit they would have 'intentions to force a woman to sexual intercourse' if nobody would ever know and there would not be any consequences, a shocking new study has found."

"Nearly one in three college men admit they might rape a woman if they knew no one would find out and they wouldn't face any consequences, according to a new study by researchers at the University of North Dakota."[25]

Here are the facts:

Three researchers—Sarah Edwards, Kathryn Bradshaw, and Verlin Hinsz, two from the University of North Dakota and one from North Dakota State University—published a paper in 2014 in the journal *Violence and Gender*. Their paper was titled "Denying Rape but Endorsing Forceful Intercourse: Exploring Differences Among Responders." The topic was excellent and the methods seemed appropriate for the seventy-three male students who completed a survey, attended a debriefing, and completed all the other parts of the study. All the young men were over eighteen; over 90 percent of them were white; all identified as heterosexual; and all claimed prior sexual experiences.

Go back and read the news items: "1 in 3 men would rape a woman if they could get away with it . . . "; "nearly one in three college men admit . . . "; "close to 1-in-3 collegiate males . . . "

In other words, these providential seventy-three young men ended up standing in for the entire male population. Not just in North Dakota. Not just on college campuses. Not just in the world today, but in all history. The researchers themselves were far more modest in their claims. But enough of the popular press ran mock-shock articles that it's worth asking why. Reading these news accounts, you could be impressed by the new scientific evidence that rape is what a lot of men want to do, especially if it's not called rape: more men will rape if they can be assured of no future negative repercussions. If there is threat of punishment, stigma, and shame, numbers of rapes will be kept lower than they would "naturally" be.

Certainly, press outlets want readers and will often stoop to fudging the truth and sensationalizing the news. More than that, however, there were underlying assumptions these news items could mine and exploit. Saying one in three men would rape if they could get away with it tapped into preexisting beliefs; many people believe that regardless of class, or region, or race, a lot of men want to rape women. Sure, they called it rape culture. But the news coverage made rape culture awfully like male culture, and male culture dovetailed awfully easily into underlying beliefs that more men would if they could. The problem with picking up on a tiny study from North Dakota and turning it into screaming headlines read by millions of people goes beyond lax editing standards: it spreads confusion about men. Who gains in this instance is actually not easy to determine.

Rape is not just any bad thing, and debate about why rapes occur has become ground zero for the range of views and experiences with gender and violence overall in our societies. The science of rape, or rather, the scientists of rape, tell us that rape is natural in some preordained way. That is the only way to explain, they say, that rape is found everywhere and always in history. Why men rape is a central question of our time, however, and we have to get it right.

Even though numbers around rape are notoriously hard to come by, what numbers exist are by general consensus underestimates by an order of magnitude. In the United States, according to a Centers for Disease Control study from 2011, one in five women and one in seventy-one men will be raped at some point in their lives. Moreover, 46.4 percent of lesbians, 74.9 percent of bisexual women, and 43.3 percent of heterosexual women reported sexual violence other than rape during their lifetimes. One in four girls and one in six boys in the United States will be sexually abused before they turn eighteen years old.[26]

Rape culture is not unique to the United States. Rape is found in every region of the planet, and accounts of rape are among the earliest in human records. But rape culture is stronger in some societies than others. One of the foremost scholars of rape, Peggy Sanday, explicitly links the incidence of rape to the "overall position of women" in a society. In places where women have significantly more power and authority, rape cultures are weaker. In places where interpersonal violence and male dominance (in governing, business, and culture, for example) are more pronounced, rape cultures are stronger. Sensationalist news accounts that only partially digest and present the findings of scholarly studies can too easily grab readers' attention because of preexisting beliefs, which then does more harm than good in limiting rather than fostering complex conversations about maleness and masculinity.[27]

MEN WITH BALLS

It was 1970 in the United States, and the Vietnam War was raging. So were massive social movements around black liberation and women's rights. Richard Nixon was president, and the majority of citizens not only favored the war effort, but strongly opposed the upsurge of demands from a significant but definitely outnumbered contingent of protesters of all stripes. The line of demarcation between Republicans and Democrats, conservative and progressive politics, was not as clear as it might later become. Though the Republicans had a more consistent record of opposing women's rights and feminism, the Democrats were all over the place, a chaotic political umbrella concealing incompatible viewpoints, strategies, and programs. The Democratic Party presidential candidate in 1968, incumbent vice president Hubert H. Humphrey, defeated the progressive wing of the party represented by Eugene Mc-Carthy to become the nominee before getting a drubbing by Nixon in November.[28]

In July 1970, Humphrey's personal physician, Dr. Edgar F. Berman, used his bully pulpit as a man of medicine and science to warn his fellow Democrats against the folly of choosing women as leaders for the party or the nation. Dr. Berman was a retired Maryland surgeon, a member of the Democratic Party's Committee on National Priorities, and a newspaper columnist. His rationale was squarely biological as he ticked off possible dangerous scenarios: a "menopausal woman president who had to make the decision of the Bay of Pigs"; a bank president "making a loan under these raging hormonal influences at that particular period"; and a "slightly pregnant female pilot" making a difficult landing.[29]

Berman's thoughts on the high rates of alcoholism, obesity, and heart disease among male CEOs and politicians, to say nothing of Woodrow Wilson's stroke, Dwight D. Eisenhower's heart attack and ileitis, John F. Kennedy's Addison's disease and back problems, or Lyndon Johnson's gallbladder operation, all while in office, were not shared at the time. And there is no way he could have predicted the effect of Jimmy Carter's excruciating hemorrhoids on the Iran hostage crisis.

In case anyone thinks that men declaring women incapacitated from leadership on account of menstruation debilitation is a thing of the distant past, an obsolete relic of a bygone era, recall the infamous words of Donald J. Trump when he explained why a female television anchor had asked him tough questions: "She gets out there and she starts asking me all sorts of ridiculous questions, and you could see there was blood coming out of her eyes, blood coming out of her . . . wherever." Why else? This was forty-five years after Berman cautioned his Democratic colleagues against admitting women to the top ranks of the party. Many were outraged at Trump's flagrant sexism, but why? His logic was consistent with widely held ideas about women and their cycles.

What is supposedly inevitable in women, their animal natures, is exactly what makes them ineligible for office, in this view. Men's animality, on the other hand, is what makes them the right kind of raw material for political leadership and state-sanctioned forms of violence. But really, in both cases we are dealing with moral evaluations, not biological facts.[30]

Or take another case of violence: What if I walk up to you on the street and shoot you dead? Most observers would agree this would be homicide, justifiable or not. But what if I am the president of the United States and I send you to fight, and you kill for your country? Does that make me a murderer? Or an accessory to murder?

When officials of the United Nations use the term "intentional homicide," they are distinguishing different kinds of killing, and specifically excluding what they call war- and conflict-related killings as "socio-political violence." These can include hate crimes, which are products of social prejudice. Whether "gender-based killing," based on sexual orientation and gender identity, should be considered intentional homicide or sociopolitical violence remains a bone of contention.[31]

The issue is more than the loophole distinction between killing and murder. What is it like to grow up as a man in El Salvador or South Sudan or the Philippines in an era of society-wide armed conflict waged by militaries, paramilitaries, and civilians? For that matter, what does it mean to grow up as a man in the United States in the first part of the twenty-first century, at a time when the country invaded and occupied and waged endless wars in the Middle East, when its armed forces were stationed at a thousand military bases stretched across the globe, and when torture was officially sanctioned for use against designated enemies? What impact did foreign incursions, combat, conquest, and overall hawkishness have on boys as they grew into men?[32]

We have become too accustomed to linking certain kinds of violence with men's physiological capacities, to thinking that men are more prone to aggression of all sorts than women. When violence is on a small scale, interpersonal and domestic, it is widely deplored. However, when violence is used by the leaders of nations in wars they say are in defense of freedom, democracy, and national sovereignty, then suddenly violence becomes authorized and applauded. In the United States we are only too familiar with rationalizations of state-sanctioned violence. But it is worth noting another aspect of how we think about different kinds of male-initiated violence—in particular, the symbolic distinction between prohibited and honorable violence: When men commit "bad" violence we are more likely to hear of links to their bodily compulsions (maleness, race, mental capacity, economic status). Justifications for "good" violence, on the other hand, are invariably tied to "higher faculties," cerebral functions said to manifest especially among male leaders. Then again, some do not have higher faculties:

"I did try and fuck her. She was married."

"I moved on her like a bitch."

"I don't even wait. And when you're a star, they let you do it. You can do anything."

"Grab 'em by the pussy. You can do anything."[33]

That this is the future president of the United States speaking each line has been remarked upon and decried repeatedly. The most shocking aspect of these violent threats against women is not that Donald Trump once said these things. Or that, despite listening to this wanton bragging about sexual assaults, tens of millions of women in the United States voted for him anyway. Or that none of it seemed to matter: even after boasting about physically attacking women, Trump still got elected. We're not talking simply about people who unashamedly countenance violence against women. There were plenty of Trump supporters who oppose those kinds of attitudes and actions. They could nonetheless vote for Trump because they were willing to overlook his sinful behavior and were able to rationalize those words and deeds as unfortunate consequences of being a male leader. There was, in other words, complicity in the acquiescence, and that collusion was rooted in bedrock beliefs about men and women and violence.

A button popular in the 2016 US presidential campaign read, "VOTE TRUMP: Finally someone WITH BALLS." The real-world consequences of such unsubstantiated claims are painful. Trump was elected not despite his repeated remarks championing sexual assaults on women, but because of them. He was chosen to lead because tens of millions of people in the United States believed that boys will be boys and that those who disagree should get with the program. In this view, the sins of Trump are simply those of untethered masculinity in its original form.

While by no means exclusive to men in power, blatant misogyny among elites can shed light on the more pervasive problems linking men, power, and essentialist thinking. Focusing briefly on China, for example, by the 2010s, earlier rhetoric about the goal of gender equality in that country had all but disappeared from most government proclamations. But that didn't mean that it was absent in leadership discussions. Political guidance seemingly unrelated to men, women, and gender in recent years has been raised by China's leaders in a remarkably gendered fashion.

In 2012, the same year he became the secretary general of the Chinese Communist Party, Xi Jinping gave an internal talk to party leaders that was soon dubbed the New Southern Tour speech. In this talk, later released for the general edification of 89 million cadres, the secretary general insisted that the economic and financial reforms throughout the country must continue, and must be led by the Communist Party, but that the leadership of the party should effect these societal reforms without reforming the party itself out of existence. In particular, he cautioned the Chinese leaders that they should learn from and guard against mistakes made earlier in the Soviet Union during its period of broad reform. One of the central headaches facing Xi was how to maintain the leadership of the party in a Chinese capitalist market economy and society that had experienced one major reform after another in the previous decade.

Xi's talk concluded with a pithy provocation meant to drive home his point that the Chinese could not afford to follow in the reformist footsteps of their erstwhile brethren: "In the end, nobody [in the Soviet Party] was man enough to come out and resist." Not that no one was brave enough, or skilled enough, or clever enough, or determined enough. No one was man enough. Around this same time, another Chinese leader, Major General Luo Yuan, complained about the moral decline of China's (male) youth, criticizing them for growing soft when they needed to toughen up. As he put it, "masculinity and strength" were the magic bullets that could put Chinese society back on track.[34]

Injunctions from China's president to be more manly are not that different—in meaning or effect—from Donald Trump glorifying sexual assault. The 2016 US election was an assertion of male privilege and of the impunity to be enjoyed by powerful men who committed sexual assaults against women. Tens of millions of people heard Trump's statements and appreciated them for their deliberate excess. Of all the vicious aspects of Trump's pussy-grabbing comments, we should worry most about blandly accepting the idea of powerful men doing what all men wish they could in an almost effortless, depressingly banal, and supposedly authentic pursuit of man's primal needs and pleasures.

CHAPTER SIX

I AM, THEREFORE I THINK

*Today a husband's impotence is often blamed on the dominance
or carping of his wife. In the sixteenth century, it was usually
blamed on the power of a woman outside the marriage.*

NATALIE ZEMON DAVIS

ANYONE WHO RAISES LIVESTOCK KNOWS THAT YOU SOMETIMES HAVE
to keep males and females away from each other in order to control
when they breed. Segregation of male from female humans, in both
public and private venues, is remarkably common as well. For all sorts
of reasons, legal, religious, athletic, and even choral, we keep men and
women, boys and girls, apart. Even the language and symbols of separation by sex and/or gender are routinely presented as if the boy/girl
separation were the most ordinary arrangement. The binary physical division by sex is also one of the more taken-for-granted social norms—for
example, separate bathrooms for men and women. Recent challenges
by trans people, among others, have led to feverish discussions and
sometimes new ground rules and legislation, just as gender confusion
has fueled these debates in myriad ways.

Protecting women has been the rallying cry of conservatives who wish
to maintain and sometimes extend gender segregation. In one sphere after

another—from the military to sporting events to separate spaces on public transportation—studies are commissioned, psychologists consulted, and religious texts invoked to evaluate the perils of sex mixing. Central to these discussions is the question of whether women are more or less disadvantaged by segregation from men in different circumstances and whether men are fairly or unreasonably stigmatized by gender segregation in those same circumstances. If we think there is something irredeemable about men and women, that they are like other animals in some inflexible way, such that certain kinds of gender separation are necessary or beneficial, then it is fair to ask whether continued segregation by gender is an admission of defeat and a retreat from attempts to change men's behavior toward women, and if so, to what extent.

MALE BONDING AND GENDER SEGREGATION

Do you think there is some persuasive reason that men require substantial separation from women? If you're a man, do you have a strong primeval urge to spend time bonding with your buddies? If you answered yes, then you may be responding to a primordial call of the wild that goes back to before the Stone Age, when men were hunters, and hunters went roaming in male bands of brothers-in-arms. Or, maybe not. Perhaps you dismiss the cranky essentialism behind "male bonding." But that doesn't mean you haven't used the phrase. Deep down, you still may wonder whether men sometimes need to gather by themselves in groups. Don't all men need time every now and then for a little male camaraderie?

From man caves to bro-outs, it is taken usually as inevitable that men are driven to spend time without women. But a scientific justification for this idea is actually fairly new. It was originally conceived by the anthropologist Lionel Tiger, who argued that men have an elemental impulse to spend quality time carousing, imbibing, and chowing down with other men. None of this would be particularly relevant were it not for the fact that men must now figure out how to respond to the educational and occupational achievements of women. For some men, this means focusing on improving relationships with women. For others, bonding among themselves provides the best prospect for male catharsis and self-protection.

"Succinctly stated," Tiger offers, "men 'need' some haunts and/or occasions which exclude females." Through such male companionship they experience solidarity with one another. Male bonding, according to Tiger, is a trait that has developed over millennia, a process with biological roots connected to the establishment of the all-male alliances necessary for group defense and hunting, a compulsion that he believes was the same on the African savannah in 80,000 BC as it is wherever you live today. He might have had a point, aside from just one tiny hiccup. Evidence from the bioarchaeological record indicates a remarkable "evolution of hypercooperation" between men and women as well as a "pervasive ethic" of "sex egalitarianism" when hunting and gathering were the main forms of existence for humans. Indeed, there is good evidence that until the advent of agriculture some 10,000 years ago (the dates vary by region), when animals became more scarce, hunting was more of a joint effort by men and women together.[1]

One of the underlying assumptions in the theory of male bonding, whether rooted in evolutionary theories or not, is that there is something logical and commendable about segregation by sex. In the United States, the term "segregation" reasonably makes us recoil in horror; we think of *Plessy v. Ferguson*, the 1896 "separate but equal" Supreme Court decision, and all its later consequences. But consider instances in which segregation is widely accepted—such as in medical quarantines, with their separation of the sick from the rest of the population in cases, for example, of tuberculosis; here, segregation is a recognition that the infection can spread and needs to be contained. Segregation doesn't mean there is no cure, or if there isn't one yet, that you won't look for one.

And as gender studies scholars have long recognized and taught, there is nothing automatically unequal and unfair about gendered divisions of labor, with one gender group having more responsibility for certain needs, for example, and another group assigned to other needs. To the extent that these divisions of labor—you do the kids, I'll do the cooking—reflect not hierarchies and power imbalances but more efficient ways to organize tasks, such as care for the young and provision of food, we talk about gender complementarity.

But what about instances of segregation that do contribute to social inequalities, either because a persecuted sector of the population is separated to make their situation worse (*Plessy* again), or because segregation in the name of righting wrongs can instead exacerbate problems the separation was intended to confront?

By even considering that male bonding could be embedded as an indispensable male requirement, we create reasons to believe that there are other ways men and women should be separated socially and materially in the modern world. How much we actually know about men's exclusive communications and male-only enclaves is debatable. We certainly notice male-only spaces for their gender segregation. But simply noticing is not really analyzing why they endure. Is there a relationship between men's secret houses in New Guinea and men's clubs in New York City? Chicago taverns and Athens coffee houses? What about sports arenas in Moscow and gay bars in Madrid? Video parlors in Timbuktu and Tacoma barbershops? We are certainly aware of them, but I'd wager we don't spend much time reflecting on persistent male-only segregation more than to disparage or defend it.

Humans employ gender segregation in a variety of ways for multiple reasons. In the case of patriarchal societies, it is not hard to see why institutionalized support for men-only spaces, such as private clubs, can be tenacious. Only in 1984 did Harvard College sever formal ties with its notorious male-only "final clubs." For well over a century, young men who went on to fame and fortune in politics, the arts, and business made early and lasting social connections in these semi-secret societies. A list of a few of the notable men to grace these mansions in Cambridge gives a taste of their importance—and if you have to ask who they were, you clearly wouldn't belong: from the Fox Club, T. S. Eliot, Bill Gates, and Henry Cabot Lodge; from the Fly Club, no less than Franklin and Teddy Roosevelt, Oliver Wendell Holmes, Jay and David Rockefeller, and Jared Kushner. (In 2016, Harvard finally announced sanctions against the male-only clubs still in existence.)[2]

In the United States and other countries, male-only institutions are where important discussions are held and decisions made in private. The idea that such men just need a little downtime with other men once in a while is a fig leaf used to justify the exclusion of women who want access to power. These all-male settings shape and reinforce insidious forms of masculinity. And because the activities in these clubs remain hidden from public scrutiny, they can remain unquestioned (and even unknown) by women and other men who would find them abhorrent. Women are kept out to stifle their attempts to mount challenges against entrenched male dominance.

Whatever the motive—to exclude women from key male domains or to get some me-time with the dudes—such "homosociality" has social and political consequences that can't be truly understood by looking at nucleic acids and proteins, aka, chromosomes. If we invent the idea that men have certain physiological needs that they do not in fact have, we are basing our attitudes about gender segregation on false premises. Perhaps women don't need to be protected so much after all, and men don't need to be protected them from their own bad selves. Biobabble about men and sex, and men and violence, leads to bad social policies, or at least incomplete attempts to resolve serious challenges like sexual assault. To the extent that we consciously or unconsciously buy into the idea that men are controlled by their bodies, that they think with their dicks, that their thoughts and actions are somehow beyond their ability to control—that the way men come prepackaged in fact controls them and how they think—we concede defeat to gender-based violence and a host of other social dilemmas.

In public policies the rubber hits the road in the science of maleness, gender confusion, and beliefs about male animality. In 2016, the

North Carolina state legislature passed House Bill 2, or HB2, the so-called Charlotte bathroom bill. Officially known as the Public Facilities Privacy and Security Act, the law reversed an ordinance that had extended some rights to gay and transgender people and nullified local ordinances around the state extending protections to LGBTQ persons.

HB2 had little to do with bathrooms. Instead, it was an assault on LGBTQ communities in North Carolina and nationwide passed by a legislature obsessed with genitalia and sex. For those who know US history, of course, segregated bathrooms are nothing new. And segregating bathrooms on the basis of race is obviously racist. Why has there never been an outcry about separate bathrooms for men and women? We all take this separation as equitable and reasonable, the only real debate being who qualifies to enter the different bathrooms. What is it about urine and feces that is so remarkably different in men and women that their evacuation needs to be done in separate spaces?

The history of gender-segregated toilets in the world seems driven by the entry of large numbers of women into industrial labor, in Europe beginning in the nineteenth century. With more women in the workplace, accommodations were built for their exclusive use. In many countries today, the "urinary leash" continues to be an issue, meaning that if there are no available bathroom facilities for women in public areas, women are more likely to be bound to their homes. Obviously the vast majority of people in the world, where separate bathrooms are available, have become accustomed to this kind of segregation, and even if they can accept trans people using whatever bathroom they are most comfortable in, there are few people clamoring for everyone to be able to use the same bathrooms.[3] Yet comfort and custom here are directly based on nothing more complicated than genitalia and the social strictures that make genitalia a decisive feature, one that comes with its own taken-for-granted restraints.[4]

There has been similar public debate about occupational segregation, and the arguments in this debate, too, are rooted in competing perspectives about the biological differences between women and men.

The furious deliberations in the United States and other countries regarding whether to open combat positions to women in the armed forces, touched upon earlier, are but one example. These debates focus on the question of proximity, segregation, and how close is too close for men and women in uniform. In January 2013, Secretary of Defense Leon Panetta nullified the standing policy that did not allow women in units "tasked with direct combat." Worries persisted, however. One worry was about men and women falling in love in the trenches (apparently it happens all the time); others concerned inappropriate fraternization, or the psychological cost to male soldiers when they witnessed women getting wounded or killed.

Even the poster child for alleged gender equality in the military, Israel, is far less integrated than it might seem at first glance. Israeli women serve shorter stints than men. Although technically they are allowed to serve in 90 percent of the roles in the military, they actually serve in only two-thirds of the positions. Women in Israel can receive exemptions from military service far more easily than men and avail themselves of these opportunities far more often. Furthermore, as one authority on the subject reports, "the Israelis have consistently refused to put women in combat since their experiences in 1948," because at that time "they experienced recurring incidences of uncontrolled violence among male Israeli soldiers who had had their female combatants killed or injured in combat." In this instance, "I am, therefore I think" gets translated into men who can't control themselves from brandishing their innate protect-the-women bona fides if they get too close to women.[5]

Segregation is a recurring theme not only on the battlefield, but also, of course, in many religious doctrines. Among the more discussed gender divisions are those found in branches of Judaism, especially ultra-Orthodox and Orthodox Judaism, where rabbis are always men, women are always separated by a *mehitzah* partition in religious ceremonies, and various other rules apply to only women or only men among the faithful. Adherents believe this kind of segregation preserves gender "modesty" and assures attention to prayer, and that it is only through the physical separation of males and females, particularly during religious ceremonies, that these aims can be achieved.

These rules have received attention in the press following encounters on international airline flights, especially from the United States to Israel, when some ultra-Orthodox men have refused to sit next to a woman to whom they are not related. Flight attendants and airlines have had to handle these incidents carefully; meanwhile, it can cause flight delays and stir controversy. Not all ultra-Orthodox men insist on such seating arrangements—it's difficult, if not impossible, for single travelers to arrange ahead of time for a certain seating arrangement, beyond "aisle" or "window"—but enough have insisted on male seating that it has become a periodic news item. Airlines have pushed back against this kind of separation, but the underlying religious motivations remain the same.

Sometimes in these incidents, women passengers agree to switch their seats with another passenger, typically with help from a flight attendant. So I am less concerned here with what some ultra-Orthodox Jews want and why they want it than with these passengers' decisions to acquiesce. What is involved in the thinking of these generous passengers, who cede to a male's demand to move so that he won't have to sit next to them? They are not just showing courtesy, but implicitly condoning the premise that a man, because he is a man, cannot sit next to a woman because she is a woman. If a passenger said, "Because of my faith, I cannot sit next to a Jew," no one would have a hard time dismissing this person as anti-Semitic and showing him the nearest exit. Why is it different when a woman is asked to move? Is there an underlying belief that it is not so outlandish that a man who is a total stranger could nonetheless react to some irrepressible urge when in the vicinity of a woman? That notion is objectionable, maybe, but not implausible.[6]

Presumptions about men's underlying nature don't have to be particularly complex or grounded in scientific findings. They can still influence our private and public lives in ways we take for granted. Our overreliance

on biological explanations for men's behavior can have significant repercussions. Whether segregation by gender contributes to a problem or is a
remedy to a problem is worth debating.

WOMEN-ONLY SPACES ON PUBLIC TRANSIT

In Germany, Korea, China, and other countries around the world there
are designated "women's spaces" in parking garages and elsewhere to
help protect women from assault. Women-only subway cars are common in public transportation systems in cities such as Rio de Janeiro, São
Paulo, New Delhi, Tokyo, Jakarta, Cairo, Shenzhen, and Mexico City.
In Germany, a regional train from Leipzig to Chemnitz began assigning
women-only compartments in 2016; some passengers welcomed the option, while others thought it was a step backward. In several cities with
women-only subway cars, feminists have taken to the streets and subway
platforms to protest the segregation and to demand that men who prey
on women, on subways or anywhere else, be apprehended and punished.

To what extent do our perceptions about maleness and femaleness
shape how we think about protecting women from men? To the degree
we abide the notion that "men, because they are men, are tempted
to assault women on the subway if they think they can get away with
it," we might allow preconceptions about maleness and femaleness to
guide public policies. There is no doubt that we need public policies
to contend with sexual assaults by men against women on subways. But
for many of the cities listed above, the idea of using women-only buses
and subway cars, especially during rush hours, as a solution to the problem of sexual assaults on public transportation has been fraught. Cordon men away from women, or at least provide women the opportunity
to separate themselves from men: Is it an enlightened decision, or a
step backward?

You might look at the cities with women-only subway cars and
think, "Brazil, Egypt, India, Indonesia, China, and Mexico. The global
South seems to have more problems of sexual assault." We could also

look at the list and think, "Maybe the global South has better solutions to sexual assault." Gender segregation on public transport in Mexico City, for example, has been popular with transportation planners and women riders, though it has been criticized by some feminists for not adequately addressing the roots of men's assaults on women. At the heart of the debate is the question of whether men are coded by biology to prey on women, and the most that can be done is to quarantine them away from women, or men can be stopped, punished, or changed. And there is a short-term and long-term discussion as well: some argue that it's a necessary measure similar to affirmative action in the United States, remedial and necessary for a time, a temporary way to safeguard women until the behavior of enough men is reformed. Others say that such pragmatic policies can too easily detract from the real effort that is needed to fundamentally confront and stop male sexual privilege and assault.

Six out of ten women who ride Mexico City's public transport system have experienced some kind of physical or verbal assault. Only Bogotá is more dangerous for women getting around the city on buses, subway cars, and jitneys. Perhaps even more extraordinary than the statistic that hundreds or even thousands of women are accosted daily in Mexico City is the debate surrounding what should be done about the problem. The discussion revolves around implicit attitudes toward men and sexual assault and why men do these things. Or, rather, why some men do them. And, in addition, how the authorities can stop them. Disagreements about solutions reveal deeply held beliefs about how to develop transportation strategies in response to men abusing women.

In 2008, the Mexico City government created the ATENEA program, named for the Greek goddess Athena, to prevent, apprehend, and punish sexual violence against women traveling on public transportation. One result was the expansion of a system already in place called "Solo Mujeres," which included spaces on subway cars and buses designated for women only and children under a certain age. Elderly men are sometimes allowed there, too. As of 2017, the program was still being expanded to incorporate more trains on more lines during rush hour, as well as the newer Metrobus lines in the city.

Although the program hardly resolves the problem of men molesting women on the Metro cars, it was effective enough for many women to take advantage of the opportunity for self-segregation. Yet the program's expansion has not been accompanied by any developed analysis of what is causing problems of violence on public means of transportation to begin with—whether it is all a matter of men and sexual violence, or humans and violence, or some other mix of unidentified factors. This analysis has not been elaborated because it doesn't have to be: without needing to be told, we all know what is involved and why, right? We all think we understand the reasons for violence on subways and buses without having to conduct a study. When women complain of pushing and shoving by other women on the women-only cars, it might seem anomalous; we do not equate this, in any case, with men's sexual assaults on the mixed-sex subway cars. We assume these are not the same kinds of violence.

Women-only spaces on subways and buses help, but they do not resolve the underlying problem of men molesting women on the Metro. Still, despite the shortcomings of these measures, many, and probably most, residents of the capital, women and men, support this kind of gender separation when it is feasible on public transportation. The fact that men can enter women-only cars at Metro stops where there are no police to stop them, and, of course, the fact that separation creates new issues for women who are traveling with men on the Metro, are secondary considerations—frustrating, but not enough to negate what many women see as a necessary measure to protect them. Although sitting in the women-only cars is voluntary for women, and some of them, at least in Mexico City, choose not to use them, the program is of practical importance. It has measurably improved female riders' safety, and it serves as a symbol and a constant reminder that a problem that could be taken for granted is being addressed.

The residents of these cities do not necessarily think about the problem in terms of whether men (and women) are controlled by their bodies, or whether men's thoughts and actions are ultimately reducible to biological, chemical, and material processes functioning in their brains and genitalia, or whether someday we will be able to predict people's ideas and actions through the physics of their brains, and perhaps prevent those brains from causing bad things to happen. And yet what is really being disputed is the extent to which we as societies are in a profound sense controlled by the ubiquity of men's bodies and their influence over societal decision making and policies in ways large and small, in everything from government to business to family matters. If men's bodies hold these particular threats without even trying, then whether you call it the Realm of the Y Chromosome or the Estate of Testosterone, it spells trouble for societies until it is recognized, accepted, and contained.

The Solo Mujeres program entails more than providing women with separate spaces and preventing men from entering those spaces. The alternative to mixed trains also conveys a very pointed message each time a woman gets on the subway at rush hour. Walking by signs, or even by a walled-off corridor, a woman is plainly reminded that she can receive certain protections from men clawing at her, making rude comments, and threatening her. Simultaneously, however, the separation sends a message to men: you are forbidden from entering those cars. Every time a man gets on the subway at rush hour, he is visually and tangibly reminded that he is not to go on specially marked cars, and why he may not enter those women-only havens. If he has half a wit about him, he is compelled to think again about the reasons for the separation of men from women, to consider what actions could have led to isolating men from women, and perhaps even to determine whether it is women being sequestered away from him, for their own protection, or him being quarantined off from women, because as a man he might be dangerous.

There is a contradiction latent in the fact that in case after case around the world, men's desire to segregate themselves from women is most often aimed at enhancing men's own pleasure and prerogative. When women are segregated, whether by their own choice or by social edict, it is more commonly aimed at protecting women from men.

The ATENEA program in Mexico City has always sought to provide safe, comfortable, and inexpensive transportation services for women, and its public announcements promote free service for pregnant women, the elderly, and those "with different capacities." When I interviewed Martha Delgado Peralta, the former secretary of the environment for the city, she admitted that ATENEA still had not yet been able to resolve the core problems: the groping, pawing, and need for child protection on the Metro system. She drew two diagrams for me, one showing everyone stuffed onto the same car, and the other with separate cars, one for men and one for women and children. She added a timeline, arbitrarily choosing a five-year endpoint in the future. To meet that target, Delgado told me, men would need to change to such an extent that women-only subway cars and similar kinds of gender separation on public transportation would no longer be necessary. In other words, gender segregation on public transportation should not be a long-term situation, she said; it was an expedient measure she hoped and expected would not always be necessary.

The biggest challenge Delgado and other authorities face, however, is not setting a deadline, or even developing an agenda to raise public awareness of the problem of sexual assaults on public transportation— no one who regularly uses the subway could possibly be unaware of the concern. The bigger obstacle is ingrained thinking about men, temptation, and access, and whether anything can be done beyond trying to prevent men from doing what comes naturally.

What measures would Delgado propose that could be instituted to change men? Here she seemed less convincing. Could we only hope to change the expression of men's urges? She raised the idea of vigilance: riders could report problems to Metro teams, and teams could then nab molesters red-handed. She was optimistic that men could be changed, though, because—here she stopped to point to a bicycle behind her in her office—hadn't she changed the mindset of residents of the capital when it came to biking? Hadn't people warned her that there was too much dangerous traffic in the city, and no bike culture in Mexico, and that biking would never catch on? Well, she informed me, there were now bike lanes all over downtown Mexico City and new bikers all the time, thanks to her efforts to change people's attitudes and practices around biking. Changing men so they would not assault women would be a similar challenge, tough but achievable.

I talked at the end of 2014 with another city government representative, Saúl Alveano Aguerrebere, who had coordinated the program to integrate Mexico City's transportation systems. He thought maybe people were overthinking the problem of men accosting women on the Metro. If we treated men more like the children so many of them still are, we could cope better with the problem. Just separate them from others, exactly the way one does with fighting children. He wasn't kidding, either. When a responsible government functionary says the solution to the problem of sexual assault by men against women in any context is to treat men like children, the message is akin to boys will be boys. An offhand quip becomes state policy. That's shocking, but what is worse is that our reaction to it—when we hear that a government official has said we need to treat abusive men like children and separate them when they fight one another—may be to concur with a resigned nod of agreement.

In Mexico City, as in other cities across the globe, when faced with the crisis of sexual assaults by men against women on subways and other means of transportation, a major social problem, government authorities came up with a partial way to address the problem, and then set to work implementing the stopgap solution. Who besides abusive men could oppose this arrangement? As it turns out, some feminists. Their reasons speak directly to the question of our underlying assumptions about men, sexuality, and violence. Even for people who don't call themselves feminists, there are some thoughtful concerns about the women-only spaces.

PROTEST AND THE SEMANTICS OF ABUSE

The politics of the women-only Metro cars on the Mexico City subway are manifest in the language employed to describe the problem these cars seek to address. My friend the radiator repairman, Roberto, lives an hour and a half from his workshop in the neighborhood of Colonia Santo Domingo, where I used to live. He spends most of his three-hour-long daily commute on the Metro. I asked him about men, women, and sexual assaults on the subway. Roberto suggested that we distinguish between "assault" and "touching."[7] I told him I thought he might be missing the point.

If the former meant harassment, molestation, and assault, whether physical or verbal or both, the latter for Roberto meant simply to touch, to come into physical contact inadvertently, an action that invariably happens on a crowded subway car. Touching happens because of circumstances beyond anyone's control, but assault is caused, he believes, by "culture" and "education," meaning here not so much formal education as upbringing by parents. Roberto was sure that better child-rearing could significantly reduce assaults on the Metro. He agreed that it makes a difference whether one is pushed by a man or a woman, and whether it was a man or woman getting pushed. For a woman, even if you are getting crushed by others inadvertently, it isn't fun, but it's not the same as when a guy pushes against you with his shrimp. Words to live by.[8]

Although I have some middle-class friends who use the Metro, by and large the Metro is for working-class riders who may not have an alternative means of transportation. But even for those in the working class, the subway is not for everyone. I met my old friend Delia when we were first neighbors on Huehuetzin Street in Colonia Santo Domingo, a rough-and-tumble area deep on Mexico City's south side. She and her family were among the squatters and land invaders—the local word is "parachutists"—who descended on the area beginning in September 1971. Like her husband, Marcos, Delia worked for decades cleaning up classrooms, hallways, and offices at the nearby National Autonomous University of Mexico, UNAM. Both Marcos and Delia are used to physical challenges, including the gangbangers who are as much a part of the fabric of the community as they are.

The words they use to describe violence of various kinds, the people they hold responsible, and the situations they describe shed light on popular perceptions of how much about violence can be tied to men and maleness, and how much to poverty and hustle, or to infrastructural factors that are present in Mexico City, such as overcrowded subway cars. Their language of engagement with social problems, including violence, reveals underlying assumptions about causes and solutions, too.

But when it comes to the Metro, Delia says, she'd rather not even go. She'll squeeze into surface road jitneys and buses instead. "The Metro scares me," she told me. I admitted that, despite the injunction above the doors in subway cars—"BEFORE ENTERING LET PEOPLE EXIT"—I, too, have been scared of the scrum getting on or off the train at certain stations. The question then arises again as to the difference between violence and gender-based violence. Should we distinguish between these categories, and if so, how? Women like Delia may see violence as pervasive in the world, and they will want to do whatever they can to avoid it no matter who is inflicting it. But they also may have trouble seeing the women-only cars as a significant step forward. Riding the Metro still often requires sustaining bruises and worse from women riders. For a woman who has seen her fair share of men beating women, Delia is never reluctant to pin blame on men when it's due. But her frightened assessment of the Metro is of a generalized violence rather than an especially gendered violence.[9]

The point is not to provide travelers' advice, a guided tour to the troubles and violent tribulations of the subway system in Mexico City, but to ask how violence is described, understood, and adjudicated in the minds of citizens in that city and others like it. For Delia and other women, men *are* animals sometimes, but so are women. For her and others in her neighborhood, violence is extensive and relentless. But she would say it stems as much as anything else from scarcity and hardship on the lower rungs of society. This view might be something to consider, especially in contrast to the more gender-based rationales for the women-only subway cars and buses. If this alternate view seems like a description and explanation that blames the poor, Delia might agree.

It is not just Delia: many of her neighbors also trace the causes of violence not so much to every man's predisposition as to other social factors. And some of them look farther up the ladder of social success and power. When I asked Doña Fili, my oldest friend in the neighborhood (we met in the summer of 1991) what she thought of the women-only Metro cars, she spoke as if the subway system had a mind and body of its own, "El Metro es agresivo, Mateo," she cautioned me: the Metro is aggressive. The aggressiveness of the subway stemmed not from a male-only problem, in her view, but was a product of too many people being forced to cram into too few spaces. For Fili it was a matter of class oppression as much as anything: the poor ride the Metro because they cannot afford cars as easily as the better-offs. And the Metro capacity is nowhere near sufficient to serve the needs of the poor. If there is violence and aggression, it comes from those in government, the financial sectors, and other powerful entities who make the decisions that affect how the poor will live.

If you ask her, Fili will tell you that she is opposed to splitting up men and women on the Metro. In fact, she is dead set against it. Fili, a community activist in Christian base communities, in neighborhood associations, and in citywide political movements, sees the mere existence of gender separation on the Metro as tacit acceptance of male assaults, the authorities essentially giving up the struggle against a widespread social ill. If men prefer to stand in solidarity with women and in opposition to men who assault women, Fili wonders, how does separating the men from the women help? For her, masculinity is not a congenital disease.[10]

The sharpest critics of women-only subway cars are Mexican feminists, who argue that to endorse this kind of separation by gender on the Metro cars is to capitulate to bad behavior, a declaration that the government officially believes men can be restricted but not changed. It does nothing to address the root causes of men sexually abusing women. After all, the city would never have a special car for riders who wanted to be free of pickpockets—they prosecute other types of crime, so why not this one? These social critics insist that men who are abusive must instead be stopped and punished, not simply separated from women.

Doña Fili opposes the women-only subway cars because she thinks men can change. Fixing the problem, for her, is a matter of changing men's attitudes toward women, and she believes that needs to start at the top. Once, in 2000, when she attended a presentation for a book on what it meant to be a man in Mexico City, Fili stood up and challenged the mainly academic audience not to think machismo was something just in poor families and neighborhoods. Look at the political party that had ruled Mexico for some seventy years, she insisted. That's where you'll find the *real* machos![11]

For many people, if not Fili, the women-only subway cars and other measures, such as capturing and prosecuting offenders, can happen hand in hand. Would women feel safer as a result of both measures? Informal surveys indicate that most would. The central concern must still be less about the immediate, most apparent causes of sexual assaults on public transport, less about the local debates, and more about a fundamental issue in Mexico and across cultures worldwide: What do we expect of men, and how do we meet those expectations? What spaces should they be allowed into, and where should they be excluded? Unless we understand why men assault women, we may be appalled, but we will not be surprised when it happens on public transportation and people continue to assume that we cannot hope to change a thing about it.

As part of a campaign against sexual assaults on subways in Mexico City, UN Women (that is, the United Nations Entity for Gender Equality and the Empowerment of Women) and the Mexico City government launched a campaign, #NoEsDeHombres, in 2017. The advertising agency J. Walter Thompson beat out forty competitors to win the bid

to raise public awareness around the issues. In one sensational intervention, a subway car seat was transformed so that it resembled the front of
a man's body, modeled in such a way that if you sat down on it you were
forced to sit on the man's penis. A plaque on the floor in front of the
model read, "It's a hassle to travel here, but it's nothing compared to the
sexual violence that women suffer in their daily travel."[12]

In addition to the penis chair, there was another avenue of attack
through videos, including "Experimento Pantallas," with tight shots of
men's derrieres displayed on public screens for all to see. The idea was
to force men to see what it feels like to be leered at. The bottom line for
the campaign overall was that men were the problem, and that women
already knew this, so what had to be addressed was men's resistance to
acknowledging their complicity in sexual assault against women.[13]

TOLERANCE AND MEN MIXING

For those in favor and those opposed to the women-only cars, the larger
issue raised is whether you want to treat the symptoms of male assault or
actually want to cure the illness, says a young man I know, Miguel. I've
known Miguelito almost as long as I have known Doña Fili, since 1992,
when he was four years old. As we talked about the women-only subway
cars, he told me that for him, the main issue was whether we could
preach *tolerancia* when it comes to men who assault women. We could
not be forgiving of these men. They had to be reeducated about why
assault was wrong. Miguel had grown up in a family of strong women,
in a neighborhood with strong women leaders. He could not accept
that tolerance approach. To do so was to say that we had to accede to
prevalent ideas about men and sexual assault, that there was something
normal about sexual assault. Miguel seems constitutionally opposed to
that approach.

Political theorist Wendy Brown has written effectively about the
same word Miguel used, "tolerance." Usually in political discourse this
term is associated with liberal thought. But Brown notes that although

many liberals hold tolerance in the highest esteem as demonstrating an openness to the ideas and habits of others, there are limits to this philosophy. If tolerance is your highest goal, and the most accommodating approach you can think of is to incorporate and accept a wide range of beliefs and behavior, you can inadvertently foster forms of discrimination that you mean to oppose.[14]

No one, least of all Wendy Brown or Miguel, is saying we should tolerate sexual assault. But to the extent that we think we have effectively regulated sexual assault on women by providing them with separate subway cars, we might also be implicitly tolerating sexual assault in other contexts. For instance, it might seem to be acceptable on mixed subway cars, in packed escalators, on stairs, and in the corridors of the Metro stops. In other words, Miguel might have been closer to the truth than he realized when he criticized the idea that we should show tolerance toward men who assault women. Even if we support safe-space cars for women on subways as a good move, we need to caution against the tacit message that any woman who chooses to ride in a mixed car must accept the risk of sexual assault.

Public policies always aim to improve the delivery of effective social services, including addressing needs that arise from gender inequalities, abuse, discrimination, and the like. When policies relating to gender inequities are developed in one locale or another, one state or another, or one country or another, implicit assumptions about men and women invariably creep in with little or no open debate. Gender segregation may seem like a good way to attend to matters of women's safety day to day. Yet at what cost do we build such policies without taking a more critical view of how our premises address the needs of men and women? The cost of not asking the deeper questions—or, really, of continuing to develop policies based on our faulty presumptions, with respect to sexual assaults on women, for example—is to slip into the problems Wendy Brown calls out.

Many people take it for granted that men and women should be separated in particular places and times. Consider the example of bathrooms again. When we take the seemingly innocuous division of male/ female for granted, what happens is that people—and in the contemporary world, that means especially trans people—get hurt. Tolerance is beaten back with specious legal rulings. Or consider again religious practice that involves gender segregation. It's one thing to say that membership in a religion is voluntary, and thus people accept such separation as part of participating in the organization. But when the requirements of religion spill over into public space, things become more complicated. Even the kindness of strangers on planes can contain seeds of unavoidable collusion with certain ideas about men and their primal urges when they are around women.

Seen from this perspective, we can look once again as well at our earlier discussion of conscription. In addition to essentializing the violent tendencies of men, the continuing practice of registering and/or drafting only young men can be seen as another instance of a public policy based on fallacious beliefs. These beliefs about men—that they are violent, and more suited than women to war—remain unexamined and unchallenged, and instead simply and uncritically accepted as reasonable and ordinary. If we see analogous patterns in other policies, relying on similarly unquestioned assumptions about men—say, concerning men in business, or men in tech companies, or men in government—it will become apparent that such policies are not just rooted in local ideologies and cultural practices but grounded in more widespread tenets of faith about men-as-men.

Why is there virtually no opposition to regulations about young men alone being registered for a possible future draft? Perhaps it is because we are perfectly comfortable accepting that young men and young women are by nature fundamentally different when it comes to violence. Why is segregation by some religious groups broadly accepted, or at least ignored, but segregation by other religious groups vilified? These differences show how gender separation ultimately reflects social and political standards more than anything intrinsic to male and female bodies. Whether in public or private, the exclusion of one group or another carries a language of division and difference. Though these may not be bad in themselves, it is certainly worth considering whether the separation is justified or might perpetuate inaccurate representations.

If physiological male/female differences are the motherlode of pseudoscientific thinking about sexual assaults, sexual temptations, and gender segregation, then the evolutionary El Dorado is the range of behavior shared in common by all animals: parenting. We all know parenting is as social as it is individual, that parenting styles and values vary from family to family and culture to culture. What we think about fathering in all its guises and disguises will reveal a lot about what we think about men, evolution, and maleness.

CHAPTER SEVEN

FATHERING

*Perhaps there are still children who
have not eaten people? Save the children.*

Last entry in "Diary of a Madman" by Lu Xun

I N THE MID-1970S, POET ADRIENNE RICH FAMOUSLY DISTINGUISHED the difference between fathering and mothering. "To 'father' a child suggests above all to beget, to provide the sperm which fertilizes the ovum," she wrote. But "to 'mother' a child implies a continuing presence, lasting at least nine months, more often for years." In the time and place Rich was writing, her understanding of fathering and mothering might have been appropriate, and not coincidentally it dovetailed neatly with popular understandings about the parenting habits of other animals—for example, how traits like "maternal instinct" were common across species. The question for us is whether what she says is always and automatically true. Are mothering and fathering fixed or flexible?[1]

Alternate definitions of parenthood have always existed. But we often tend to view the world through a lens of our own cultural making, so it's easy to forget that men in different cultures father in different ways.

The phrase "traditional dad" can slip off the tongue as a way to describe our own fathers or friends. Terms like "traditional" or "modern" or "usual" or "unusual" are all used to modify fathers, to tell us something important about what one person does in comparison with others. Yet what people mean by "traditional dad" is likely to vary quite a bit. A father who is especially protective of his children could be said to be traditional. But then so could a father who abandons his children. Or, if not "traditional," exactly, maybe such a father might be seen as "typical" in the eyes of some: the point is, it rarely seems as surprising or shameful when a father neglects his children as when a mother does. A father who is especially tender is acting like a traditional father, as is one who is particularly strict. A father who roughhouses with his children is traditional, as is one who is more distant from them. A father who is never around, and a father who is always around, might both be called "traditional."

Writing about a small agricultural village in Mexico in the 1940s, anthropologist Oscar Lewis described fathering as a distinct set of experiences that men had with their children, especially boys, while they planted and harvested maize, chiles, and tomatoes. "The father assumes an important role in the life of his son when the boy is old enough to go to the fields," wrote Lewis. "Most boys enjoy working in the fields with their father and look forward with great anticipation to being permitted to join him. Fathers, too, are proud to take their young sons to the fields for the first time, and frequently show great patience in teaching them." Historically in China, as in Mexico, during the harvest seasons a boy of six or seven was expected to learn "by trying to work within sight of his father." And in China, as elsewhere, the pattern for centuries was that after a next child was born, "the older child begins to sleep with his father instead of his mother. . . . When this change occurs, the father begins to dress the child, too."[2]

The idea that modernity finally challenged a "traditional" way of behaving in which fathers had nothing to do with children until the current era is absurd and ahistorical. It serves no purpose other than to make people feel good about men who do more with children than their (similarly urban-origin) fathers did. When men moved to the cities from the countryside, and began working in factories or driving buses or selling items in the street, they left behind not only their oxen and plow but also their ability to father in an intimately engaged fashion every day of the week. Much about what seems "traditional," and in this sense "natural," in terms of parenting divisions of labor reflects more about modern myths of the past than about ancient truths as to the kinds of interactions fathers and mothers had with children of various ages.

When we talk about "traditional dads," whatever that might mean, it becomes shorthand for whatever has been replaced by some other pattern of fathering. If we scratch the surface of fathering and mothering, we find not only tremendous variation across cultures and historical contexts, but, perhaps most significantly, generational shifts. The differences in parenting across generations belie our belief in common features of fatherhood that we supposedly share with other animals. Unique to humans, patterns of fathering can and do change dramatically in a short period of time.

IMAGINARY FATHERHOOD

I went to a cocktail party in an upscale neighborhood of Mexico City many years ago, ferrying my two-month-old baby in a Snugli *canguro* (literally, kangaroo). A man introduced himself to me as a banker and remarked, "You know, we Mexican men don't carry babies!" He told me that's why he made money, so someone else would carry his babies, change their diapers, and care for them until they got to "the age of reason." But in the squatter settlement where I was living at the time, a lot of Mexican men did carry babies and young children, and they were not disparaged for it.

Back in my neighborhood of Colonia Santo Domingo, when I repeated his remark, it was met with disdain. "That's silly. Haven't you seen the guy who sells vegetables at the open market on Saturdays? The one who keeps his baby in a cardboard box under the table?" The banker's statement sharpened my awareness of some striking differences based on class, resources, and values within the Mexican capital, especially related to who thought fathering involved more than making a baby.

As it happened, three years before this, in 1989, I had been walking through downtown Mexico City when something caught my eye through a doorway. I turned back, focused my camera, and took a picture of a man holding a baby while talking to a customer in a shop for musical instruments. When I later showed the photo to friends in Mexico and the United States, I got rather consistent responses: "That can't be," was the gist. "We know Mexican men are machos, and machos don't carry babies." All I could say in response was that I had taken the picture in Mexico, and I assumed the man was Mexican.[3]

I decided to carry a copy of the photo with me during fieldwork in Mexico City and to informally survey people's thoughts about it. It ended up being a photographic Rorschach test. "Is his woman sick? His face looks like he's suffering." "He must be *indígena* (Indian), because *mestizo* men wouldn't be caught dead like that." "That photo is *irreal*. My husband never carried our kids." "Please don't show that photo in your classes; that's not the way Mexican men are." "That baby must belong to his boss who made him watch the child." These comments were all from middle- and upper-middle-class people, most with liberal, feminist politics.

In Santo Domingo, the responses were the opposite. The most common response I got from neighbors was, "Seems normal to me." Not every man there carried babies and toddlers, but many did, and no one found it odd. This was clearly a question of class. To some degree, the poorer you are, the fewer options you have, including with respect to family divisions of labor. So who has which duties in Mexico may be more fixed in families with more resources. You could even say that rigid gender roles are a sign of privilege. But we all know this is not really true, as women from the working class do more at home than their husbands do, whether the women are also working outside the home for money or not. Still, class sometimes matters in unexpected ways. Among more working-class couples in the United States, for example, a prevailing ethos is often that men should work outside the home and women within, but in practice they share duties more than they say or think they do. In the middle class it is often the opposite, as husbands and wives assert they both share household chores a lot more than is the case.[4]

After collecting responses to the photo of the man in the music shop over a period of four years, I decided to solve the mystery behind the man with the baby. I couldn't remember exactly where I had shot the picture, but after walking around for a couple of hours downtown, I eventually walked by a doorway through which I saw a wall of mandolins displayed. I realized I had stumbled onto the place again. I went inside, took out the photo, and, feeling a bit like a detective in a murder whodunit, asked a young woman behind the counter, "Do you know this man?" Much to my surprise, she shouted out, "José, come quickly, it's you! Some guy's got a picture of you!"

José Enríquez came out from the back, without the mustache he'd had in 1989, but possibly wearing the same shirt. Finally I would learn the truth. I told him I had taken his photo many years before, and, feeling increasingly awkward about what I was saying, tried to explain why my obsession with his picture had led me to spend years studying fathering in Mexico. Fortunately, José was a patient man, and he kindly explained that the baby belonged to a neighbor who lived upstairs from the shop, and that the mother sometimes left the baby with him when she went out shopping—"It's so much easier to shop if you're not carrying around a baby. Besides, I was not going anywhere, and I like babies." He shared a photo of his own three children, and then he asked me gently, "Don't men like babies in the United States?"

INHERITING SINGLE MOTHERHOOD

Over the years my friends and neighbors in Mexico City have taught me about what they see as the importance of genetics to understanding why fathers and mothers do what they do. My young friend Daniel is an unusually sensitive guy. I've known Dani since he was born. When he was a teenager he painted large, lush portraits based on religious iconography that still hang proudly on the walls of his parents' home. Because of his early devotion to the world of ideas, his graceful demeanor, and his deep wellspring of caring for others, his mother, Norma, thought Dani might become a priest. I am always struck by his delicate take on the world.

Yet the world around him has not always been so gentle. He has lived all his life in the neighborhood of Santo Domingo. Dani knows women who are well represented in community-wide associations. Women who are key to block organizations. And women who hold their own in household discussions and decisions. But he also knows how uneven and unsteady change sometime seems, with one mother and wife leading marches on municipal authorities downtown, while her neighbor has to ask permission from her husband to leave the house.

I was back visiting the neighborhood and explained that I was thinking about the relationships between gender, culture, and biology. Dani said he thought families and communities were obviously important influences, but there were some things only biology could explain.

"Do you know Gloria, the single mom who lives down the street?" he asked.

"Yes," I answered.

"And you remember that her mom is also a single mom, right?"

"Sure."

"Well, did you know that Gloria's grandmother was also a single mother? And her great-grandmother? And her great-great-grandmother, too?"

"I didn't," I told him.

"So, okay. It's one thing to say that one or two generations of single moms is a question of culture. But when it's *five generations*? At that point it has to be hereditary."

Dani was raised in a settlement of land occupiers of Mexico City, with poor families and poverty all around him. He had made it to high school, where most students have to take general biology. Genetics is a component of that course, in Mexico City as elsewhere. This means all students who finish high school in the capital are at least exposed to basic ideas about genes and their powerful ways. Just because Dani studied genetics doesn't mean he thinks that biology explains everything. But at a certain point, he believes, you just have to admit that it matters. Dani was visibly pained by the suffering of these women and their daughters. He was not dismissing their predicament: biology provided a way of showing mercy for the women. Ultimately Dani was saying they could not help themselves from becoming single mothers. It was in their blood. This was not a superficial and unconcerned analysis, but heartfelt empathy sharpened by high school genetics textbooks.

Yet what a panoply you can find when you get beyond contemporary assumptions in those textbooks about men's supposed compulsion to sire more children. There are the "milk fathers" in poor areas of Brazil, who provide store-bought powdered baby formula for the mothers of their children even when they are not otherwise active as fathers; the "left-behind father-carers" in Indonesia, who pick up the slack to care for their own children when their wives, the breadwinners, emigrate to follow work opportunities outside of the country; the paternal "gestures of affection" among Palestinian fathers tending to their hospitalized children; the "check fathers" whose only fathering is financial. In parts of the Caribbean, men with many children have long been known as having "strong blood." In China, parents to this day quote the ancient philosopher-sage Mencius, who said, "There are three ways to be unfilial; having no sons is the worst."

The famous anthropologist Margaret Mead developed a test she called "the negative instance": all you need is one exception to a particular theory about the way all humans are, and you have in effect eliminated biological determinism as an explanation for that behavior. If we apply this test here, all we have to do is find "negative instances" for uniform patterns of fathering to conclude that culture is key, that biological programming is less consequential than we often assume, and that change is possible.[5]

Context is everything. Other patterns of fathering may seem foreign; it's a good thing when we are astonished by them. It's good to hear, "Well, maybe that's the way fathers are there, but that's not the way we do it in Moose Jaw, Canada." Or Ganja, Azerbaijan. Or Stepaside, Ireland. Furthermore, if we have our sights set in any way on shared parenting by men and women, and equality of responsibilities, and investment in children, it will all seem less daunting if what we aim for represents a break with mere centuries of habit—or maybe only decades—rather than millions of years of evolution.

MIGRATION AND FATHERING

Talcott Parsons, one of the most influential social scientists of the twentieth century, tracked modernity's progress in the 1950s by an increasing, not decreasing, social division of labor, especially within the family. For Parsons, the ultimate familial achievement lay in the realization of distinct duties, with mothers finally able to specialize in their collective and biologically mandated task of child-rearing and men devoting themselves to more outside, public pursuits. Adrienne Rich's analysis about the distinct meanings of "fathering" and "mothering" did not come from Parsonian modernization theory, but it revealed widespread attitudes that often reflected less the realities of actual fathers and mothers than the societal standards in vogue in influential academic and government circles.[6]

One of the consequences of migration and urbanization in Mexico, and the new, modern division of parenting labor, was the development of a new form of child neglect that goes under the name of *mamitis*, or mommy-itis. This folk diagnosis reflects the influence of biomedical ideas about children's expected demands on and attachment to their mothers as well as the increase in women's obligations regarding child care following the rise of urbanization in Mexico. This psychological childhood trauma, often mentioned in a humorous way, has always been dependent on socioeconomic as much as subjective factors. As grandmothers left behind in the village became a less viable option for parents in cities, and child care woefully lacking for many working parents, *mamitis* was used as an excuse (by both women and men) for women not to work outside the home for money. It was also a form of protest against the transformations demanded of modern families. The concept is comparable in many ways to what psychologists in the United States might call separation anxiety, or being a mama's boy (or girl), except that it was taken out of the realm of the interpersonal and made a reflection of social dislocations especially impacting women as mothers.

Mexico is not alone: child care has changed around the world in recent decades. But these changing patterns reflect socioeconomic factors more than they prove an evolutionary link to parenting practices. In many of the changes we see a direct impact not just on women and how they mother, but also on men and ways of fathering. There are, to date, no recorded case histories of *papitis*, however, and this means that in societies around the world men are often less expected to be good parents than was the case only fifty years ago. Their presence as active participants in child-rearing is not seen as being as important as it was in recent memory.

My older daughter, Liliana, spent her first year of life in the squatter settlement of Santo Domingo. When she started eating solids I would go to a butcher shop down the street because the shopkeepers, Guillermo and his brother, would grind up meat twice when they knew it was meant for an infant. As I was leaving one day I shouted back to thank Guillermo, and I said, "Okay, gotta go home to cook this up with some pasta and . . . " Before I could add, "some vegetables," he interrupted me and scolded, "No, not pasta. That's just going to make her fat. You know, Mateo, that the father doesn't just procreate; he's also got to make sure they eat right."

The need for men to take a crash course in how to feed children has become a major issue in recent decades across Southeast Asia, where the "feminization of migration," both internal and international, has led to the widespread phenomenon of "left-behind fathers," mentioned earlier. These fathers shop, cook, feed the children, bathe them, launder their clothes, and tell them stories at rates never before witnessed in recorded history. Categories that have long naturalized the stature of fathers and husbands as the masculine pillars of the home alongside the assumed association between women and nurturing have been undermined by the need for greater earnings and the work opportunities available for women as guest workers abroad. The feminization of migration has challenged age-old God-sanctioned and Confucian-based models of family hierarchies—precursors to modern naturalized frameworks of fathering and mothering—in Indonesia, the Philippines, Vietnam, and other Southeast Asian countries.[7]

In roughly two-thirds of families in Indonesia and the Philippines with a mother absent for most of the year to earn money for the household, the stay-at-home father is the primary caregiver for their children. In other homes, grandmothers and other relatives pitch in, though some complain that grandparents are such "soft disciplinarians" that it's better to leave children in the hands of their fathers. Unsurprisingly, some people, fathers and others alike, have an easier time adjusting to new duties and identities than others. For some men in Southeast Asia, assuming household and child-rearing responsibilities is a way to prove their ability to solve problems, provide materially for their offspring, and otherwise prove their masculine strength and ability to overcome obstacles to achieve whatever they set out to do. Others are bothered by issues of emasculation and inadequacy, given their wives' greater earnings, and it can be hard to ignore these concerns. "No money, no power," intone some men, who nonetheless may reasonably claim that they, too, continue to contribute materially, often through agricultural income.

Researchers report growing numbers of men expressing greater sympathy for the household tasks their wives have shouldered since time immemorial. In fact, these tasks take on an increasingly degendered hue as men cook meals, bathe the younger children, and look after every other aspect of daily family life. Their lower economic status compared to their migrant wives means they also often have reduced decision-making power, at least with respect to major investments and purchases. Revealing the contradictions of the age when it comes to defying hallowed gender norms, one Vietnamese woman who left her home in a village in the Red River Delta, to work in Hanoi, remarked, "My husband is the master of the family, but I am the decision maker. He is the pillar of the home so that our children will see our model. If I want to make a decision, I make it, then inform my husband before we implement it."[8]

For most of the twentieth century, a protracted struggle for gender equality has unfolded in many areas of the world. These have involved suffrage, reproductive rights, education, work opportunities, and campaigns against gender-based violence. Modern, reliable, accessible forms of birth control have transformed our intimate lives. Migration is no longer a demand placed on men alone; indeed, the feminization of migration has forced dramatic changes in the lives of fathers and children. Feminist political movements have both responded to and propelled these social disruptions. And simultaneously with these tectonic shifts, even as biology is assigned an ever more controlling presence in human actions, men and women throughout the world have been renegotiating maleness and masculinity—what it means to be a man, and what it means to be a father. Some are even considering whether fathering and mothering might one day mean the same thing.

In a study of psychiatric training in the United States, Tanya Luhrmann, a psychological anthropologist, writes of "a moral vision that treats the body as choiceless and nonresponsible and the mind as choice-making and responsible." This moral vision entails signaling whether the humans who happen to inhabit male bodies have fewer options in controlling their actions, such that it would be less useful to hold them accountable, and whether the best we can hope for is to find effective mechanisms to contain men in their uncooked form. There can be few issues more sensitive to mind-body distinctions than fathering: beliefs in fathering as synonymous with procreation alone are really just dressed-up versions of saying men are nonresponsible bodies, that we would do best to expect little from them in the way of child-rearing, and that we should be pleasantly surprised when they manage to break free of their corporal compulsions.[9]

MY COUSIN RICHARD, THE EMPEROR PENGUIN

"Over 95 percent of the world's more than ten thousand bird species are raised by two attentive, hardworking parents," writes ornithologist Richard Prum to help ward off unrelenting human-animal comparisons that exculpate fathers who are largely absent in rearing offspring. Why else do we regularly encounter flabbergasted articles in our daily newspapers about the same animal species—seahorses, pipefish, emperor penguins, smooth guardian frogs, and marmosets, to name a few—where the males defy standard reproductive practices? For example, in the case of seahorses, fathers give birth instead of mothers; with emperor penguins, the male alone incubates the egg, while with other kinds of penguins males and females take turns incubating.[10]

My cousin Richard defied gender and familial expectations when he and his wife, Audrey, decided before their first son, Andy, was born that Richard would be a stay-at-home dad. "The idea that Audrey would have stayed home with the kids was never on the table," he told me. "She really liked the working thing. I also think there was probably a feminist aspect to it. She wanted to go out and prove something. She's really good at what she does. I probably wasn't as good. She had all the fancy credentials [like clerking for a Supreme Court justice]. I was always more interested in staying home and taking care of the kids."

When did his sons realize they had a strange caregiver situation? "I was super-involved in their lives," Richard said. "I don't know if that's a good thing or a bad thing. I would always sign up to be the Room Mother. I coached the Little League soccer team. I was the swim coach. I'm sure I embarrassed the hell out of them sometimes. But it was all they knew. Besides, Andy's best friend also had a stay-at-home dad. He's an aspiring screenwriter and adjunct professor of film. He basically stayed home and his wife's a doctor. So maybe the boys didn't see this arrangement as all that strange."

Richard reports that when some people heard this was what he did "for a living," the response was sometimes, "Really?!" But mainly he heard, "Wow! That's really cool." He thinks that if he'd been a woman and said that he stayed home with the kids, they would have been far less impressed. One friend told him she thought his two boys were probably more independent because of the arrangement. He demurred, telling me, "I don't know if I'd agree with that because I probably have too many female traits in me." Besides, Audrey was a lot more involved in raising their sons than the average male partner in a law firm would have been. "I don't know whether that's some kind of maternal instinct or because culturally moms feel they need to be in on it more, or what," Richard said.

The hardest challenge was how to tell his father (my uncle)—who, like Richard and his two brothers, was a lawyer—about his decision to leave the bar and devote his life to raising his children. "I think he was a little bit in shock," Richard said. "He never expressed disapproval, but I was afraid to tell him, thinking I would be disappointing him. Our grandfather was very successful in the business world. My father was successful as a lawyer in ways easy to measure. I never felt like I was letting the kids down because I wasn't putting food on the table." I interrupted and told him that, indeed, he literally had put food on the table. Richard continued, "The idea of breadwinner was never an issue. But the idea of a career, of being preeminent in your field, was something I never got to do."

Early on, Richard was tempted when the law firm where he had worked before called and asked him to return. His mother—my aunt, and a stay-at-home mom with yet another law degree—agreed to help out with the kids, telling him, "The first six months are critical in a child's development. So even if you walk away from it now, you've done something significant." But he decided against returning to work. "Having one person, the mother or the father, stay home makes life and marriage easier," he said. At one point, he and Audrey sat down to take stock of how this unusual arrangement was working out for each of them and their two sons. "And I told her I thought I was taking advantage of her," Richard said. "She was having to work so hard to put bread on the table. And she said, 'I feel like I'm the lucky one. I can always just do my job and when I come home there's always food.'"

I asked Richard if he thought his sons, one now out of college a few years, the other just finishing, might follow in his footsteps. "Would either of my boys be a stay-at-home dad? I really doubt it." Change comes hard. Maybe Richard would say that only a man who has—as he put it—"too many female traits" would stay home to cook, clean, and care for the kids. But I'm pretty sure he would be comfortable with the idea that becoming a stay-at-home dad is a matter of being able to afford it, individual temperaments, and a couple's overall aspirations for their family. Richard is a compassionate person, something you can see in his interactions with others; in other words, he has a quality thought stereotypically to be a maternal one. He is also someone who, by staying home, has long been bucking the system. There is something wrong with our thinking if compassion is seen as a consummate female trait and bucking cultural traditions is not.

GENERATIONAL SHIFTS

If biology were more determinant of fathering patterns, we would expect to find great uniformity across cultures and historical epochs, and we would not expect to find rapid change in fathering patterns from one generation to the next, much less one year to the next. The very particular case of Palestinian fathers who leave occupied Gaza to take their children to Israel for cancer treatment, however, highlights just how tenuous gender divisions of labor can be in the contemporary era. Caught up in political currents beyond their control—living in territory occupied by Israel since 1967, with borders closed in 2001, and a blockade emplaced in 2007—families desperate for decent medical treatment for their children stricken with cancer have few options.

The most common decision in these Palestinian families is for the mother to stay home with the other children while the father accompanies the ill child to a hospital in Israel. Once there, according to one recent study, the father faces the difficult and disorienting challenge of having to place his trust in the medical personnel, who not only do not speak Arabic but are assumed to be hostile to Palestinians in general. Whether at home in Gaza or in a Tel Aviv hospital, "the Israeli-Palestinian conflict is the prime factor shaping the lives of Gaza fathers." Fathers were already expendable at home. They were available for the task of taking the child to the hospital because their labor was already chronically underutilized. But the transition to providing "maternal" child care is not nearly as problematic as some might imagine. By taking on this role, the Palestinian fathers inadvertently unveil the "fragility of gender roles, and possibly also some of their arbitrariness," according to the study's authors.[11]

The political exigencies of life in the Palestinian territories force families to adapt and often to make creative decisions concerning gender divisions of labor, including, in this case, with desperately ill children. That fathers and mothers have consistently and quickly bent the culturally proscribed, gendered rules is testament to a quality of human adaptability shared with no other animal. Their example attests to the limited importance of biology in determining actual fathering practices. Widespread patterns can develop in human societies based on biological differences—notably pregnancy and lactation—but they are mere evolutionary pressures and not decisive or permanent restraints.

In 2018–2019, I worked with a team of practitioners and scholars on the issue of young men's sexual and reproductive health in a borough of Mexico City called Venustiano Carranza. As part of the project, we interviewed young men and women about their lives, their families, their sexual histories, their dreams for the future, and the ups and downs they had already experienced inside a sprawling, marginal section of the Mexican capital. One recurring theme in the interviews was father-hood: specifically, a number of youths talked about fathers who had abandoned them and their families.[12]

"I was barely in second grade when my mother discovered that my father had been deceiving her and she ran him off," said one young man. "For two years I saw him every Sunday, then it was one Sunday yes, one Sunday no, and now the fact is that I don't see him. Not even a message. He doesn't get in touch for Christmas or my birthday. I try to talk to him again, telling him, 'No, no, whenever you want.'"

Another interviewee told us, "Unfortunately I have a father who's responsible, but he lives with someone else, he has another partner, and another son with her. He's like 100 percent with them and like 30 percent with us, 30, 40 percent with us." Some of them didn't really know their fathers. "Well, I don't have what you could call a relation with him," one said. "I don't remember him. It's been so long since I've seen him, I don't really know what to tell you about him."

Sometimes the mothers seemed to be the main obstacles in the way of ongoing relationships with fathers who no longer lived with them. "At first it was tough," one young man recounted, "because at first I couldn't see my father. The truth is that I love him and I loved him. I couldn't see him because my mother prohibited this and that. I was always with him, from an early age. He was the one who taught me how to do things. But most of the time I spent with my mother. I was almost always with her." He laughed when he told us, "You could say I had *mamitis*. Not like now. Now I hardly speak to her."

Learning these life histories of young men in an area of Mexico City was dispiriting, but not nearly as depressing as conversations I had with my team members, most of whom were also from Mexico City. When I asked them if they thought the young men's acute awareness of their experiences with irresponsible and absent fathers meant that they themselves would be different kinds of fathers in the future, I was met with an immediate and emphatic, "No, Mateo, they will repeat the same patterns; they, too, will abandon their wives and children. That's just what men do."

I was aghast. And then I thought about it more. For young men in Venustiano Carranza to not become their fathers will depend on political and social pressures, some of which can only be guessed at. The jury is surely still out. Generational changes in fathering depend on changing men and masculinities. And changing fathering might depend on changes in women and mothering as well, and the direct, indirect, and residual influences that women have on men and masculinity.

In 1951, the English pediatrician and psychoanalyst D. W. Winnicott invented the term "good enough mothering." The concept championed the idea that when a child realizes that their good enough mother won't and can't satisfy every need, this helps the child to better adapt to the realities of life. Since then, others have extended the concept to "good enough parenting." But it might be worth further considering what "good enough fathering" might look like in the future. Just as my cousin Richard was the beneficiary of praise and support for his fathering, in part simply by virtue of the fact that he was a stay-at-home man, so, too, in the modern age men receive accolades or opprobrium based in good measure on what the speaker thinks is normal fatherly behavior, which invariably is less than what one would expect from mothers. Even to compare "good enough fathering" to "good enough mothering" can bring into relief the lesser social expectations of men with children. An exception to this rule was manifest in a simple question from a dear friend and neighbor of mine in the squatter settlement of Santo Domingo in Mexico City.[13]

As I dropped off my then four-month-old daughter, Liliana, with her *abuelita*, Ángela, one afternoon in 1992, Ángela asked me, "Is this the greatest love you've ever felt?" I told her that it was certainly different from any kind of love I'd ever experienced, mumbling something I'd learned years before about how the classical Greeks differentiated kinds of love, *agape* and all that. Ángela responded, "Yes, but isn't it the deepest love?" I told her I loved Liliana more every day, but that I was still not used to being a father. I kept expecting someone to intervene and tell me I had to give her back. All I can say is that the look on Ángela's face that day was the most awful mix of pity and disappointment (or horror) at my inability to discover and release what should have been my instinctive feelings of parental love.

Before Ángela died, I returned with Liliana for a visit and was finally able to report that the love I felt for my daughter, the fatherly love that Ángela insisted I should have possessed from the beginning, had at last and without doubt deepened into the greatest and deepest love I had ever experienced.

Change is possible.

CHAPTER EIGHT

REVERTING TO NATURAL GENDERS IN CHINA

*The Utopia of this century—that which has been
desired above all else, and desired most deeply—
has been the modernization of body and soul.*

CARLOS MONSIVÁIS

PERHAPS NOWHERE IN THE WORLD HAVE CULTURE AND NATURE been put to the test in recent decades more than in China. Say what you will about Maoism, if you come from a country that has never managed to pass a piece of legislation called the Equal Rights Amendment, the idea of at least lip service from the government for full gender equality might seem refreshing. In the most horrific days of Maoist upheaval, women and men in China were declared equal juridically and socially, and generations of women saw notable improvements in their educational, social, and economic expectations.

THE REASSERTION OF MALE PREROGATIVE
(AND FEMALE ACQUIESCENCE)

Achieving gender equality in education levels and job assignments was official policy in China from 1949 until roughly 1979. During the

Maoist period, the slogan "Women Hold Up Half the Sky" implored a generation of radical youths around the world, both women and men, to work toward societies in which gender equality was a reality. It was among the most important mantras of China's Cultural Revolution. In post-Mao Reform China—from the late 1970s on—women have been encouraged to raise and limit their sights simultaneously, whereas men have been encouraged, in official and unofficial ways, to reassume their mantle as patresfamilias. Few look back on the drab unisex clothing of the Maoist era with nostalgia—just the opposite, as ornate white wedding gowns were nowhere more popular than in China in the 2010s. But many acknowledge that at least there was the pretense of sartorial equality.[1]

Sociologists Jun Zhang and Peidong Sun write, "During the Maoist period, status and income differentials between different jobs and between men and women were relatively small." And the expectations parents had for daughters and sons were similar. After the reforms of the 1980s, anthropologist Mayfair Yang, looking back, said, "What is astonishing is the rapidity of the return of gender differentiation, the ascendancy of the male gaze, and masculine sexuality's domination of a public sphere partially vacated by the state." Gender differentiation takes different forms in contemporary China, but it always entails men realizing a greater share of prestige, power, and control at home, at work, and throughout the country.[2]

No one would claim that today's sharp distinctions between men and women, their natures and their activities, are new in China. But scholars argue persuasively that even in historical periods long ago, in which discrimination against women was widespread, the distinctions were looser than they are in contemporary China today. They did not have "the same totalizing, universalistic, and rigid essentialism that modern biology introduced into the Western [gender] binary," according to Yang.[3]

Under a 1950 Marriage Law, Chinese women won new rights, formally and often in practice, to own property, to divorce, and to exercise freedom of choice in marriage instead of abiding by arranged marriages, child marriages, and the buying and selling of women for marriage. Regardless of what women achieved after the 1949 socialist revolution, many young women in China in the 2010s were expected to reverse course. Although it is the women who have experienced these transformations most directly, men have been witnesses to them over the past seventy years. Often the targets of criticism, ridicule, and opposition during the Maoist years, more recently they have become the full beneficiaries of practices that again openly favor men and patriarchal forms of masculinity.

Between 1982 and 1998, most of the housing in China was converted from collectives to private home ownership. By the 2010s, China had one of the highest home ownership rates in the world, around 85 percent. This astonishing transformation had an immediate and momentous impact on young men and women and on courtship, marriage, and relationships with in-laws. Housing was where most of the private wealth in China could be accumulated and maintained, and it suddenly became a key symbol of emerging gender differences. In 2010, when the All-China Women's Federation and the Chinese National Bureau of Statistics surveyed over 100,000 people, they found that only one in every fifteen single women owned her own home, about 7 percent. But they found that one in five single men owned his own home, or 20 percent.[4]

For young couples who lived together but were not married, it was far more likely that the young man owned the home than the young woman. Furthermore, as private ownership of housing swept through urban areas, often only one name was required on the property deed, and that one name was usually the husband's. In case of divorce, it is not hard to see where this left ex-wives. As housing became privatized in cities, tensions intensified and became focused around a young married couple's first home.

In 2009, Gu Yunchang, vice president of the Association of Chinese Real Estate Studies, was quoted in the newspapers pronouncing,

"The rise of housing prices is due to demands from [grooms'] mothers-in-law." When pushy brides and mothers-in-law on either side were castigated for demanding apartments from young grooms, more than objectionable ideas were in play. The widening disparity between men and women when it came to property ownership—and the implicit assertion of a male birthright to own and control housing, and all new family wealth, under the post-Reform regime—was also evident.[5]

Marrying off one's child in China is related to grandchildren and is related to housing. And it's related to who will take care of the grandparents as they age. The exigencies of growing old, of eldercare, and of the new conditions in post-Reform China are connected to spreading gender chasms and "leftover" unmarried women. The phenomenon of the leftover woman has occurred despite selective abortions of female fetuses during the era of the one-child policy, as described later in the chapter, and is closely linked to the fact that these abortions historically took place overwhelmingly in the countryside, while the contemporary issue of leftover women is tied to the demographics of young women in cities and the social disruptions caused by migration and urbanization. A growing crisis in eldercare is apparent in China: old social structures and relationships that drew on collective and kinship networks are less and less tenable, or they no longer exist at all. Not surprisingly, if women decide to remain single, the care of elderly parents becomes even more problematic.[6]

In 2011, sixty years after the Marriage Law of 1950, underlying legal support for gender equality in home ownership came under direct challenge when China's Supreme People's Court took major steps to dismantle key provisions. In particular, women's property rights were severely reduced. After this point, women had far more difficulty keeping their homes after divorce, because the ruling gave explicit preference to leaving marital property in the hands of the person whose name was listed as the owner of the home. That person was almost always the husband. The 2011 decision was an important step in purging the goal of gender equality from the legal statutes governing marriage and property rights.

Women have lost ground in recent decades in China in other quantifiable ways as well. In urban areas throughout the 1970s, women's income was estimated to be 85 percent of men's, a figure that compares quite favorably to those in the United States at the same time. Following the reforms, things went in the other direction, with women's income sliding down to 70 percent of men's. Women were forced to lower their sights, and men increasingly were expected to provide the primary salary and other financial support for families. These were no longer considered joint obligations and rights in families, either juridically or in everyday practice.

China is one of the only countries in the world with a higher suicide rate for women than men. This statistic may be an indication that, despite headlines about tens of millions of bachelors in China, men have it better there. When we look more closely, however, the patterns that seem most relevant to understanding contemporary beliefs about men and their bodily components in China often adhere to urban and rural differences, and within those divisions, matters of class. In China perhaps more than in any other country in recent years, conservative, backward-looking ideas about men and their ways have been reinforced from on high and from below. Over the nearly thirty years since the state-sponsored objective of gender equality was put to rest with the reforms of the late 1970s, the gender binary has roared back with a vengeance.

But although the gender binary seems stronger than ever in China—with booming sales of white wedding gowns providing Exhibit A—that doesn't tell us why. Although some of the reasons are likely similar to those we find in other countries, what we might call the gender binary with special Chinese characteristics is remarkable for its unique qualities. Recent scholarship has pointed to several modern historical factors in its comeback.

In a country where the historical record is summoned with casual frequency in everyday conversations, at the core of understanding masculinity and femininity in China today is the need to bury the shame of the past—in particular, avoiding a return to the days of the anemic literati who proved themselves ineffectual against the disgrace of foreign subjugation during the final decades of the Qing dynasty in the late nineteenth and early twentieth centuries. Consensus on the gendered aspects of that humiliation is unanimous in China, and preventing a repeat is a commonly declared goal. That doesn't mean that everything foreign is shunned today. The backlash in the post-Reform period against the prior Maoist "cult of chastity" is intimately connected to the appeal of global cultures of gender for the middle classes. When the Chinese in the 1980s and 1990s were looking around at what the rest of the world considered modern versions of men and women, they drew special inspiration from markedly dichotomous relationships between the sexes in Japan and Taiwan.[7]

We can add to these explanations two others that have fueled and channeled the renewed attraction to the gender binary in contemporary China: one concerns the one-child policy beginning in the late 1970s; the second has to do with the failure to integrate women into the top leadership positions, despite the aim of achieving gender equality. During the era of the one-child policy, the role of the woman in the family as the (primary) caregiving parent and of the father as the (primary) breadwinner became more pronounced as a social model. As for the second factor, both historically in general and during the age of Maoism, men ran the institutions of China, including the Communist Party and its most important governing bodies—and almost every other major government entity—as well as the educational, business, and cultural institutions of the country. Modern versions of the gender binary in China are in part the product of male leaders implacably reasserting male entitlement everywhere they can. It's more complicated than that, of course, but men being in charge of everything in China is not inconsequential.

HOLD UP HALF THE SKY, OR, CRY IN YOUR BMW

Yet gender differentiation has not just taken the form of women losing rights and influence to men in post-Reform China. The literacy rate for women as well as for men went from 20 percent in 1949 to 66 percent in 1982 at the close of the Cultural Revolution. For youths, the literacy rate was 89 percent at the end of that period. Successful literacy campaigns provided a foundation for later dramatic transformations in higher education in China. Women raised their sights, and men were compelled to confront, both ideologically and in actual fact, the reality of women improving their prospects and working alongside them in field after field. In terms of educational achievements, women have maintained these advances.[8]

In other words, women have lost ground in some ways in post-Reform China, but they have maintained their progress and advanced in other respects. And this contradictory situation highlights the issue of nature and culture and gender relations: To what extent was the Maoist era, or at least the ideas espoused around gender equality, if not the actual lived circumstances, of that era, a cruel illusion, a horrific attempt to change men's and women's intractable natures? If biology is everything, then what we have witnessed since the 1970s is not so much a reversion to an unjust past as a resuscitation of predictably binary conditions, a reaffirmation that patriarchy as it has existed over the millennia corresponds to our inborn human male and female qualities. If biology does not rule gender roles, then are China's post-Reform efforts to put women back into legally sanctioned, subservient positions traceable instead to social struggles, and to different core understandings about gender roles dictated by culture? Maoism called for gender equality, but it certainly never eradicated deep beliefs in gender differences, or, therefore, enduring skepticism about the feasibility of achieving this objective.

Perhaps reflecting such sensibilities, scholarship on gender in China since the 1980s has produced mountains of books and articles documenting the rise of a new managerial class of men, both in government and business. A good portion of this work has focused on the more lurid aspects of these activities, especially the "entertaining" that new elite and entrepreneurial men must carry out to massage relationships and seal deals. From bars and restaurants to karaoke and sex, every researcher worth his or her salt has come back from the fieldwork front with sordid stories, indecent images, and narrowly escaped escapades that could compromise all but the most objective of observers.[9]

The upsurge in male bonding rituals found in karaoke bars in China means recently minted men in business suits with wads of renminbi to spend on whiskey, women, and other diversions. Anthropologist Tiantian Zheng calls the karaoke bar scene "men's triumph over women," a setting that "prepares men for triumph in the market world." The larger context for the postsocialist developments she describes is that it's "not just about a refeminization of women, but . . . also, perhaps even more so, about the recovery of masculinity." What it's being recovered from are the days of the Cultural Revolution when men were formally expected to share with women, not dictate to them, just as much in the home as in society more broadly.[10]

A widely discussed aspect of this post-Reform backlash entails endorsement or disapproval of men's extramarital sexual escapades—or simply resignation to these affairs. "Men have girlfriends," a friend informed me. "Well, not my husband," she hastened to add. "But others." There are names for these girlfriends: they are called the Second Wife, or the Little Third, and the fact that such language has come rapidly back into the mainstream of daily conversations in China suggests that it is a widespread experience, and, of course, it is always married men dating women other than their legal wives. The common expectation is that men, especially those in power, will have mistresses—and that women in power would never have lovers on the side—and the common understanding of it is that men's bodily needs were unnaturally repressed in pre-Reform China, and now can be given renewed validation.[11]

A corollary of the declaration that men need mistresses is the idea that uppity women are a problem. Men sometimes castigate the "Three-High Woman": a woman with higher education, higher income, and higher age—and therefore higher expectations. Three-High Women cannot be satisfied with the things that made their mothers happy—but they should be, according to what appears to be a growing backlash among men against women's educational and career accomplishments.

Nor is it only men who express the belief that the greater heights of society should be reserved for them. Some women, too, have quite publicly promoted the idea that what modern women want is to be maintained and pampered by modern men. In one famous incident, on a TV dating show called *If You Are the One*, a young man asked a young woman if she would be willing to ride on his bicycle for a date. Her notorious reply has been retold in China ever since: "I would rather cry in a BMW than smile on a bike." She would not be satisfied with a man unless he could indulge her every whim. For these women, for whom marriage is no longer as much an expedient with potential for romance and pleasure as an individualistic quest to meet a standard dictated by idealized gender roles, romance means little if you can't advance your material prospects. It is especially the man's role to provide a high standard of living, and if that comes with mistresses, it may be regrettable, but it's understandable if one believes that men need many outlets for their sexual impulses. That, too, fits the gender stereotype.[12]

There are contradictory pulls on young men and women in China. Some of these pulls come from parents, who have certain hopes and desires for their sons and daughters. Others come from government proclamations and policies, which can influence and constrain how people view these issues and the actions they take. Official edicts in China now rest more than anything on the notion that people must accept (and revert to) their gendered natures, thus rejecting much that seemed achievable during the Maoist era in terms of putting women and men on an equal footing. This stance contributes further to gender confusion and the erosion of gender equality. At the same time, pulls can come from unexpected directions: for example, some women refuse to accede to these reinvigorated patriarchal norms. If this contingent were to grow, it could have direct implications for ideas about men and masculinities and challenge beliefs about maleness in China that are based on popular but fallacious notions about the gender binary.

The bottom line is that gender confusion and gender renegotiation are playing out in particular ways in contemporary China in a tug-of-war between acceptance and rejection of gendered stereotypes. Do men and women have to be a certain way, or can we try to change them? Given everything else happening in Chinese society over recent decades, the renewed emphasis on male-female differences could only have been rooted in language that has the air of modernity. By looking at particular examples of the modernization of China's gendered bodies and souls, we can gain fresh insights about the extent to which the increasingly conservative gender trends in that country reflect self-fulfilling prophecies about the nature of masculinity—not just for China, but for everyone.

MEETING AT THE SHANGHAI BLIND DATE CORNER

She's not originally from Shanghai but has residence papers. She was born in 1982, stands about 5'5", has a Master's degree, and has never been married. She has a good moral character and an elegant beauty. And she has her own place to live. On the flyer her parents have posted describing her virtues at Shanghai's Blind Date Corner, we learn that she is earnestly seeking a man who is around 5'9", no more than five years older than she is, someone who is flexible as to where he lives and is willing to buy a home with her. There is no name on the flyer, just a cellphone number and the surname of a matchmaker for interested parties who wish to make contact.

Who might make that phone call? Most likely, it will be a mother or father with a son whom they are seeking to connect with a suitable young woman. And, quite possibly, neither the young woman in question nor the young man has advance knowledge that these potential connections are in the offing.

The parents in this scenario are in their fifties or sixties and come from a generation that only partially benefited from the reforms in China after 1979. Perhaps one or the other was laid off as privatization ran roughshod through state enterprises, and the Iron Rice Bowl of job security was no longer protected. These parents are also from the first generation to have China's one-child policy imposed on their bedroom. And there's a good chance that either the mother or the father, or both, migrated to Shanghai after the reforms began, part of a gigantic "floating population" of 250 million migrants from the countryside to China's cities in the 1980s and 1990s.

And now these parents find themselves separated from their village or town community, approaching old age, and left to their own devices far more than the parents from earlier generations would have been at the same age. They are reasonably growing worried about what will become of them. As isolated elders with limited access to resources, to whom will they be able to turn for assistance and comfort in their later years? In urban China in the 2010s, social safety nets were tied to residence permits (the so-called *hukou* system), and as tens of millions of migrants from the countryside did not have permission to be in the cities (even if gainfully employed), levels of social precarity for many elders became extreme. Finding a suitable spouse for a daughter or son becomes a higher priority with each passing year, for with a son-in-law comes greater potential financial stability, and with a daughter-in-law come grandchildren and the continuity of the family line. Despite the economic boom times in post-Reform China, the bottom has fallen out of life for many in the middle and lower classes. They are desperate to find a solution to their children's singleton status, and they find themselves reverting to the most basic, binary calculations of maleness and femaleness to try to resolve the conundrum.[13]

In Shanghai and in other large cities, including Beijing and Nanjing, such "Blind Date Corners" began to spring up around 2005. Aging parents and modern versions of matchmakers are the main attractions at these hubs; few children show their faces. There are certainly more parents than anyone else: they stand and sit along walkways and under trees, awaiting another parent's interest in their child's virtues. The flyers, pinned to upturned umbrellas lined up along the walkways, announce their children's best qualities. For daughters, as often as not, this is beauty; for a son, it is actual or potential earning power.[14]

There is a protocol to what information is shared on the flyers, how it's presented, and what is kept back until further contact is established. Some of the flyers look professional, complete with QR codes; others are written in longhand and include drawings, or even cross-outs and grammatical slips. They make for an endless and dizzying array stretching in every direction throughout the park. How a flyer appears is less important than its content. Matchmaker Wang told me she takes pride in handwriting flyers for her clients because she thinks passersby will appreciate the personal touch. "I really know these people," she says. Overhearing us, another matchmaker smirked and needled her: "Isn't it because you don't know how to use a computer?" she asked.

Especially on nice days, thousands of parents jostle for space, trying to score a better position in the crowd. It's a very pushy place, this Blind Date Corner, and certainly not a relaxed, genial space for idle banter about romance. Even when it's raining, or miserably blustery, or humidly suffocating, mothers and fathers shuffle along, sneaking a peak at flyer after flyer. While some might find the peddling of a son or daughter brazen, for others this is the most important obligation that parents have to their child.

They have been thrown into a precarious situation. In the big cities, it is not so easy to ensure the continuity of the family line. Nevertheless, they must succeed in helping their children find spouses, and in order to do this they must find some way of presenting their sons and daughters to the world. It was under this kind of pressure that the Blind Date Corners became popular. With brutal simplicity, even though they themselves come from a generation that epitomized gender equality and sameness (in clothing, employment, wages, and aspirations), today's aging Chinese parents tend to accentuate the most stereotypically masculine and feminine attributes, ones rooted in what they think might, just might, be preset in men's and women's bodies.

These are the parents who lived through the Cultural Revolution of 1966 through 1976, when androgyny was the tacit code of conduct, and one way they can put those days behind them is to maintain that we really should not expect the same things of men and women. The unambiguous reassertion of the patriarchy is a key feature of the post-Reform period. With it has come a re-forming of the gender binary. Prior to the twentieth century in China, kinship categories largely defined gender roles: women's identities, for example, were circumscribed by their relationships to fathers, brothers, and husbands. Biological ideas about gender binaries filtered in with scientific thinking, however, and as these notions gained ground, earlier ideas subsuming women into overtly male cosmologies began to ebb. After 1949, Maoism took on a more virulently anti-feminine guise—one reason why the backlash today includes a reassertion of feminine looks and manners.[15]

MODERN MATCHMAKERS

Parents at the Blind Date Corner can go it alone, displaying their umbrellas in hopes of generating interest from other do-it-yourself parents, or they can approach a matchmaker and pony up ¥500 (around US$75 in 2015), in the case of a daughter, or ¥100 (or as little as ¥50) for a son. In return, the matchmaker will post a flyer advertising that daughter or son for up to six months. Matchmakers used to openly set up card tables and chairs around the park; in more recent years they have had to be more discreet, as police sometimes attempt to run them off. In any case, going through a matchmaker still has advantages. A matchmaker might have years of experience in successfully finding mates for their clients' children (or so it's claimed), and may have a catalog of single young women and men to choose from (although they may or may not be real singles). The matchmakers, sitting on stools scattered along the walkways of the park, patiently going through their thick binders and iPad lists with parents with a self-assured demeanor, exude a curious blend of skills, part marriage broker and part electronic cupid.[16]

You might expect that the children on the flyers would resent these direct intrusions into what should be a subjective and private concern. And you might not be wrong. But to better understand the perspective of these young people, it helps to know a few additional facts.

Most importantly, no one—not the daughters, the sons, the mothers, the fathers, or the matchmakers themselves—wants any of this process to be called traditional. Everyone in Blind Date Corner will tell you that what is happening there is an emphatically modern event. In China, as everywhere else, what exactly it means to be modern sparks debate. People who spit, clean their noses, and shout in the public street are not modern in anyone's eyes. Yet, in contrast to Europe and the United States, religious devotion is often considered especially enlightened and worldly. Women working outside the home are viewed as urbane and progressive for some, but for others, the quintessential nouveau riche is the wife in the new capitalist supercaste, whose wealth and privilege permit her the luxury of not working for money.

Blind Date Corner is as modern as mass migration, as avant-garde as working seventy hours in an office every week. Far from conjuring the image of traditional matchmaker, the very modern realities of migration to the city and employment in office work are the most common explanations for why young people might be grateful to their parents and others who make these initial overtures with the promise of future romance, marriage, and children. They, too, want to embark on that stage of life before it's too late.

Almost every adult daughter and son in Shanghai is also acutely aware of being a single child. They were born after the one-child policy went into effect, and particularly after the state started applying the policy with greater force in urban areas beginning in the early 1980s. This generation of young people is by far the best-educated, highest-earning, and most individually ambitious group to come of age in China's long history. But it is also in some ways said to be the loneliest. Matchmaker Yang spoke to me about the crush for eligible bachelors and bachelorettes that was generated by "economic development" and "market development." To use outdated terminology, or discuss how contemporary matchmaking was related to older practices, was, he insisted, the kiss of death for business. The label "traditional" was anathema for youths caught up in the swirl of urban life.

In response to modern dating and mating dilemmas there are also new television shows in China with a large and loyal viewership. These modern spectacles include *If You Are the One, One Out of a Hundred*, or *Cream of the Crop*, along with *Luo Ji's Thinking*, with its famous moderator, Fatso Luo. As in other countries, Internet dating sites have proliferated in China, beginning in the 2000s. But parents can't go on TV for their kids, and it's creepy when they go online for them. As the Blind Date Corner matchmakers insist, nothing beats face-to-face talks, which, though taking place in a public park, seem more private. When parents beseech matchmakers to find a partner for their child, you hear anxious voices as they relate something of the child's nature and top selling points: "She's so pretty and gentle," for example, or "He's responsible and has a good car." In their intonations it's hard to miss the naturalization of emerging gender differences.[17]

At Blind Date Corner you receive a personal touch that's just not available online or on television. There are even special zones within People's Park where you can look for matches who have specific qualities. For example, there are places for Chinese prospects who have lived in other countries, such as Australia or Japan, and have returned and are open to foreigners who might be looking for a Chinese soulmate. They are all grouped under national flags in the "Overseas Corner." Foreign imports, in the form of people or ideas about manliness and femininity, add cachet and conditions to the search for a wife or husband.[18]

My favorite among the marriage mavens is Matchmaker Zhu. We've been friends since I spotted him wearing a red Che Guevara badge on his green People's Liberation Army cap in 2013—purely a fashion statement, he claimed. The niche that Zhu Wenbin has developed is to keep his clientele on both sides of the equation strictly Shanghainese, although he will offer advice to any and all who are looking for a significant other for their child. One day I asked him, "What do you look for when people come up, other than whether they are from Shanghai or among the recent arrivals?" Matchmaker Zhu misunderstood my question and thought I was asking what people should look like when they meet prospective mates: "Women should wear as little as possible, and show as much skin as possible. Guys should wear something business casual. Show their financial worth."

My friend Zhu had been no Cultural Revolution zealot, but even for him advertising women by their looks and men by their wallets in such a blatant way was a very modern twist in the matchmaking game. It was based on a salesman's knowledge of his market, which in turn was based on relapsed thinking about essential gender differences.

At the Shanghai Blind Date Corner, the intellectual and career accomplishments of daughters are generally included on their flyers, along with their physical attractiveness. Men's flyers list their height, professional trajectory, and whether they can already provide housing, along with a brief statement, written by the matchmaker or parents, vouching for their worthiness. Although some flyers at the Blind Date Corner about young women list housing as one of their positive features, it is far more likely that this information is provided for young men. The parents of young men offer the parents of young women a permanent place for their daughter to live as an incentive, and the parents of young women look for this capacity in young men. Matchmaker Zhu helped me compile a rough guide for judging the marriageability of young men and women, shown in Table 3.

One question that parents of daughters ask with surprising frequency, Zhu says, is, "Does he get into traffic when he goes to work?" They want to determine how far he lives from work and how long he will be gone on a regular basis. On a subtler level, another matchmaker, named Ling, described the ideal young man as someone who exuded confidence and elegance, someone who was more than just a pretty boy. For a young woman, even better than possessing just the generic quality of beauty, it was important to be delicate in manner and proper in conduct.[19]

Young Men/Women Should Have/Be

YOUNG MEN SHOULD HAVE/BE:	YOUNG WOMEN SHOULD HAVE/BE:
Income (ideal level variously defined)	**Appearance** (fair skinned, slender,
Work (and good prospects)	no glasses—all pluses)
Home (apartment of one's own)	**Age**
Education (equal or higher)	**Character**
Birthplace (best is Shanghai)	**Height**
Height (taller than woman)	**Education**
Car	**Work**
Age (older than woman)	**Birthplace**
	Income

Matchmakers are helping parents take the first steps not only toward marriage for their children but also toward housing and grandchildren. But parents were not necessarily out to lock their children into prearranged relationships. They merely collect the information, rather than forcing their grown children to do anything with the information they collect. "They're too busy," was the refrain on many lips in the Blind Date Corner discussions. "They don't have time to find loved ones." All the parents were doing was getting some names. Their children would make the final decision. Think of all the stress the children were being spared: they wouldn't have to start from scratch.

Perhaps these parents have too much time on their hands. Possibly a large percentage of them are retirees, and these gatherings have more to do with their own social lives than with the marital futures of their offspring. But without a doubt, parents who are panicked about their children's marriage options are overrepresented at the People's Park. It might even look like a survival-of-the-fittest moment when every Saturday and Sunday, Blind Date Corner becomes the site of earnest competition by proxy: parents armed with flyers advertising the physical, financial, and temperamental virtues of their progeny in a public declaration that they will do anything they have to in order to find a mate for their only child. As time passes without making a match, parents dig deeper into their storehouse of enticements, and these invariably embellish the most feminine or masculine attributes of their children. Despair breeds what they see as gender orthodoxy.

Despite decades of achievements in gender equality, both in China and worldwide, there is nonetheless a powerful sentiment that sooner or later men and women will revert back to their binary states. This is how people can explain other conservative pulls in China, too, like the crisis of the leftover women.

IS YOUR DAUGHTER A LEFTOVER WOMAN?

In addition to the comments in 2012 by China's president, Xi Jinping, that party members needed to man up, mentioned in Chapter 5, in October 2013 Xi urged "the majority of women" in China to double down on their child-rearing responsibilities. It was their unique duty, he said, to "educate children" and build "family virtues." Chatroom comments erupted over the clear implication that men did not need to shoulder responsibility for these duties. Some called it not just old fashioned but "defective reasoning"; others agreed that it was a "retrogression to the nineteenth century." It would be easy to dismiss the comments of Chinese leaders as antediluvian and ideological were it not for the explicit justification of their comments by appeal to the need to accept what is inevitable for men in comparison to women.[20]

Here's the thing about those flyers from the Shanghai Blind Date Corner: although it is common knowledge that in China men outnumber women in the overall population because of selective abortions of female fetuses during the one-child era, among other reasons, the Blind Date Corner operates because more women than men are looking for mates. Or, more precisely, because there are more parents looking for husbands for their daughters than there are looking for wives for their sons.

Although from the Western media you might think a key social problem in China is what to do with all the extra men who cannot find a spouse, in certain places, like Shanghai, the problem is just the oppo-

site. I gathered a random sampling of thousands of flyers posted at the
Shanghai Blind Date Corner and found the following:

- Only 35 percent of the flyers overall were for young men.
- For flyers reporting youths' salaries as "low," 67 percent were for
  young men.
- For flyers reporting youths' salaries as "high," 13 percent were for
  young men.
- For flyers reporting education levels beyond an undergraduate degrees, 29 percent were for young men.[21]

In a reversal from overall demographic trends (there are indeed
more men for fewer women, especially in the countryside), at the Blind
Date Corner there are more flyers for women than there are for men,
and the women tend to be better off financially and better educated. In
China as elsewhere, women, on average, want to "marry up," and men
tend to "marry down." That leaves men at the bottom and women at the
top coming up short more often than those in the middle. Almost 26
percent of urban women in China had been to college as of 2010, and
in fact women outnumbered men in university programs that year. The
Chinese government was quick on the case to address this very new,
very contemporary predicament, and directly launched campaigns to
correct it, sounding an alarm among the broader public that women
were educating and pricing themselves out of the marriage market.

In 2007, a couple of years after the Shanghai Blind Date Corner
began to attract customers, the all-important All-China Women's Federation issued a declaration on the "leftover woman," defined as an unmarried woman over the age of twenty-seven. The federation, decrying the
reticence of young, successful women to marry, called for a public effort
to turn this situation around, and quickly. It also began organizing matchmaking events for unmarried young women in factories around China.[22]

It might be tempting to write off the expression "leftover woman"
as hyperbole—or even as government verbiage, given the federation's

close association with the Communist Party—but the term tapped directly into mounting concerns on the part of parents of single daughters who feared their offspring could end up childless. The label exploited a deep vein of conservative thinking about the character and responsibilities of daughters versus sons. By specifying an age, and implying that the childbearing years were fast falling away, the federation's call to duty for daughters to produce grandchildren was unambiguous.

Before we attribute too much sinister intent to the Chinese authorities, we must look at the real starting point for all the fuss. Or, if not the starting point, at least the first time the term "leftover woman" appeared in print: as it turns out, it was no less erudite a publication than the Chinese edition of *Cosmopolitan* magazine. In its February 2006 issue, *Cosmo* ran an article called "Welcome to the Age of the Leftover Woman," and subsequently, several commentators have attributed the coinage of the phrase to the then editor-in-chief of Chinese *Cosmo*, Xu Wei. In China, as in the United States, if you want to know what is *au courant* in the world of gender and sexuality, look no further than the pages of *Cosmo*.[23]

Readers of the article were treated to curious claims on the roadmap leading to leftover womanhood, reflecting the intimate sociology and psychology of changing times and gender relations in post-Reform China. Soon, the "leftover woman" had made her way into newspapers and onto TV dating-game shows and sitcoms, often with a smirk, but never without a bite. Matchmaker Wang, in her sixties, with a long wall of flyers behind her, was zealous in her certainty that the leftover woman was a major challenge for contemporary Chinese society. Grinning, she goaded rhetorically, "Why is it a problem? Isn't it obvious? Why, if they don't get married by a certain age, they certainly won't be able to have babies!"

Thus was the biological clock invoked. Still, there was more at stake than mere disappearing ova. The fact was that matchmakers made catchy use of the fear of the leftover woman, insisting to passersby in People's Park that unmarried women go against nature. In many respects it represented the chickens coming home to roost on China's one-child policy, which had been launched at the tail end of the 1970s. The policy left parents feeling an unease sometimes verging on desperation. They wanted their daughter to be married. They wanted a son-in-law who could help take care of them in their old age. They wanted a grandchild. And they wanted the sanctity of marriage to be defended from the new habits of young couples living together "outside the law" and in so-called trial marriages. Relative to other countries in the region, China's marriage rates were high in the early 2000s: in 2010, 81 percent of women and 75 percent of men in China were married. And yet the fears persisted.[24]

In 2010, three years after the official announcement of the leftover woman problem, a study by the Marriage and Family Research Association, which is affiliated with the All-China Women's Federation, published the results a survey of over 30,000 people nationwide regarding attitudes toward love and marriage.[25] Of course, like political polling, surveys often not only reflect public opinion but also shape it. Nonetheless, the 2010 study is noteworthy, not least because it delineated four subcategories of leftover women (each representing an arcane play on words). Keep in mind that the average age of first marriage for women in China in 2010 was around twenty-five years old overall, and it was twenty-six and a half for women in Shanghai:

1. Women aged twenty-five to twenty-seven: "Leftover/Saintly Fighters," i.e., women who still have the courage to fight for a partner
2. Women twenty-eight to thirty: "Leftovers Who Must Win," i.e., women whose chances for marriage are dwindling and who barely have enough time for courtship
3. Women thirty-one to thirty-five: "Buddha's Leftovers from Fighting the Wars," i.e., women who have won the career wars but lost the marriage wars
4. Women thirty-five and older: "Great Leftover/Saint, Equal of Heaven," i.e., women who have it all—except for a husband[26]

The word raised constantly by parents, matchmakers, government proclamations, and on television and in print media, or on the Internet and on the radio, is "picky," as in, "Women today are too picky."[27]

PICKY WOMEN GET LEFT OVER

One man I interviewed, Matchmaker Yang, shared a variation on the picky theme, saying, "Women's expectations are too high." He thought this was directly linked to the fact that children in the late twentieth and early twenty-first centuries had so much more given to them than their parents had, and much less than their grandparents ever had; as a consequence of these better living conditions they thought they could be choosier in every part of their lives, including finding a marriage partner. Daughters had "too many requirements," starting with the husband's financial prospects, Yang lamented, adding, "Most of the time they are being unrealistic."[28]

Another matchmaker, named Chen, echoed these sentiments, explaining that the problem was that young women were too demanding when it came to young men. She insisted, "Their standards are too high." She urged young men to recognize that they have requirements that are just as important as young women's, and that they should not be so intimidated by the women that they are scared off from making contact with them and seeing where things could lead. However, there were limits, she counseled. As an example she pointed to the flyer of one young woman who listed, as one of her requirements, "serious inquiries only."[29]

Not coincidentally, *Serious Inquiries Only* is the name of a well-known television dating show. The phrase indicated to Matchmaker Wang that there was no point in even contacting this young woman "if you are even one centimeter shorter than her requirement."

Young women in modern China have been encouraged both to expand their life goals *and* to limit their goals and desires: to get a PhD, but not if it will interfere with getting married and having children; to be independent, but to find a husband who can provide an apartment for you; to have a marriage of equals, but to accept that his name alone will be on the property.

The language used in the 2010s in China to describe gender relationships—including in jest—reflected and reinforced particular, unspoken, and sometimes unconscious cultural assumptions and frameworks about the need to accept certain biological basics about maleness and femaleness. In this way, daily conversations about men and women could seem to be more an acknowledgment of unchangeable realities than an actual politically conservative campaign against women.

Daughters and sons are marketed in China by appeal to formulaic gender qualities, and the leftover women scare is fueled by anatomical reasoning. Beliefs in male-female differences are nothing new in China, but the reassertion of modern versions of the gender binary to replace official Maoist egalitarianism has required renewed emphasis on gendered biologies. No wonder a gender joke became widely told in Shanghai at this time: Do you know that there are not two but three genders in China? Men, yes. Women, yes. And the third? Women with PhDs! It didn't take long before a fourth gender was added: men married to women with PhDs.

It is unlikely that Chinese women will be returning their PhDs for sewing class certificates anytime soon. Many women are resisting attempts to strengthen patriarchal norms throughout Chinese society, but many others are trying to make the best of the situation. Men in China, as elsewhere, will either seek to benefit from male privilege or seek to break from these patterns. But to the extent that men's biological destinies—and primordial needs and presumed superiorities—are being reinforced in everyday life in China, Mexico, and the United States, the danger of naturalizing the benefits of gender birthright persists. Yet, as always, there will also be powerful countervailing currents among women and men for renegotiating maleness and masculinity. Demands for gender parity can make an equal claim to biology, in the form of new branches of the science, such as epigenetics.

CHAPTER NINE

CAN WE CHANGE OUR BIOLOGY?

There is a crack in everything. That's how the light gets in.

LEONARD COHEN[1]

BUT WHAT IF MEN REALLY ARE PRISONERS OF THEIR BODIES? WE can deplore men's sexual assaults on women and disparage deadbeat dads; we can threaten, punish, and quarantine men. But can we realistically hope to change the spots on these leopards? Maybe our only choice is to establish better social controls and admit that men cannot ultimately escape their inner sex. Maybe getting tugged back to accepting biological realities is just what we need in this era of gender confusion. Because men's biology has not changed appreciably in tens of thousands of years, it could seem foolish to look anywhere but to society and culture to address the problems that men cause. But whether biology is part of the problem or not, it certainly looks like it is not part of the solution.

One can decry the fact that with problems as varied as alcoholism, mass murder, and impotence, biology is used as a cudgel and crutch. Yet recent scientific work reveals just how much the biology of bodies and bodily processes is changeable. The discovery that bodies themselves are more malleable than we ever appreciated is bound to have dramatic ramifications in addressing social problems like male violence that were previously thought by so many, scientists included, to be more hardwired to maleness, and therefore less receptive to social influence. Some of the most exciting work in biology today is focused precisely on new understandings of how bodies and behavior interact, how organisms evolve, and how just thinking about masculinity can alter our nervous systems. More fundamentally, vulgar biological explanations for male and female behavior are especially egregious examples of pandering to common stereotypes that would ignore the past several decades of biology: confirmation of the innumerable ways the biochemistry and genotypes of all organisms are influenced by environmental factors. We should be relieved, not frightened, by the understanding that humans can change not only their cultures, but even their biologies, and that maleness is best appreciated as a product not so much of preordained laws of evolution as of very adaptable human interactions.

Accepting biological determinants outside of our control—such as ancestry—can be comforting in times of distress and despair. Men will use ancestry to explain all manner of sins. Here's a familiar example. In the mid-1990s, I did a stint in alcohol and addiction studies, including fieldwork in a rehabilitation program called the Addictions Counseling Center in East Oakland, California. One evening, as we sat in a circle of ten men, a white man who looked to be in his fifties started us off. "Hello! My name is Jimmy and I am an alcoholic." Jimmy had moved to San Francisco from Philadelphia in the 1960s and quickly fell into taking all sorts of drugs, from LSD on through cocaine. He confessed that he'd been on an alcohol and street drug bender for more than three decades. "I'm from German stock," announced Jimmy, "so I love to drink."[2]

Dennis was the next man to speak. In his early thirties, he told the group about his own addiction to methamphetamine, the restraining order his mother had placed against him to prevent him from visiting her, and his mixed admiration and jealousy of a brother's recent graduation from the University of California at Santa Cruz. He began, "Well,

I'm part German, too. And the German side of me also likes to drink."
With that, he pointed to the left side of his body. "But, the other side,"
he added, pointing to his right side, "is Indian and Filipino and can't
handle it." You have no doubt heard this kind of talk before. Jimmy and
Dennis were giving new meaning to anthropologist Emily Martin's description of people who treat "the body as nation-state."[3]

After the meeting, I stopped Dennis on his way home and told
him I didn't get the part about being Native American and Filipino,
and how this could have the opposite effect on your body and give you
a physical intolerance for alcohol. Dennis recounted that he'd seen a
program on PBS and heard that Asians and people of Asian ancestry
had a higher rate of alcohol intolerance. Compared to people of European or African ancestry, Dennis told me, this medical disorder, called
the Asian Flushing Factor, caused more people from Asia and Southeast Asia, and even Native Americans, whose ancestors had come from
that region some 15,000 years ago, to have more difficulty absorbing
alcohol. The resulting "vasodilation" (causing reddening of the skin,
called "blushing" or "flushing"), he said, was widely discussed by medical practitioners.

The problem with this thesis was that the medical literature could
only claim a higher incidence of flushing after alcohol consumption
among some populations. The idea is that flushing indicated embarrass-
ment at being unable to handle the alcohol. It's a strange claim, more
about people's psychology than anything else. The fact that this kind
of flushing never stopped anyone in China or Japan from drinking was
either unknown or irrelevant.

And more particularly in the cases of Jimmy and Dennis, if you believe biological ancestry is the card that trumps other explanations about
alcohol consumption patterns, then focusing on your genetic framework
can lead to complacency in prevention and intervention programs.

The ideas about heredity that Jimmy and Dennis shared in Oakland
revealed the influence of science programs on TV and the power of
scientific explanations to make sense of confusion about every aspect

of life, from addictions to relationships to gender and sexuality. They reached out to science—or maybe they felt as if science were reaching out to them—to solve problems, relieve despair, and find hope. They wanted to change their addictive behavior. The only way they thought they could do this was by coming to grips with what they perceived to be the biologically ethnic origins of their addictions and cravings. If they believed they couldn't change their ethnicity (and therefore their biologies), at least they could have a clearer recognition of what they were up against, and perhaps that understanding would help.

WHAT ORGAN DO MEN THINK WITH?

I was halfway through a year of ethnographic fieldwork in Mexico City when my then wife, Michelle, and our six-month-old daughter, Liliana, went back to the United States to visit family for a couple of weeks. On the street where we lived, our presence was conspicuous, and our comings and goings were the subject of widespread observation and discussion. Why didn't we just boil tap water for thirty seconds like everyone else? Was that rash on Liliana cleared up? And who was that who visited you yesterday? Where did you get that red underwear you hung out to dry on the roof? So much for the anonymity of the city. In neighborhoods like ours, it could feel like living in a fish bowl.

Michelle and Liliana left for North Carolina, and I was looking forward to a concentrated period of fieldwork and a brief break from tending to an infant who had quickly earned the sobriquet *La Cabroncita*, Little Bossy. After seeing them off, I headed to the market that was set up on Wednesdays and Saturdays under pink tarps stretching for blocks and blocks. The fruit and vegetables were fresh and inexpensive, and the sellers kept things lively. It was a great place to chat with merchants, friends, and neighbors.

Norma spotted me before I saw her. She approached, smiled at the vegetable seller, and nonchalantly asked if Michelle and Liliana had gotten off on their trip okay. I said they had. Then Norma quickly got to her point. Taking her right forefinger and placing it under her right eye, as if pointing to the eye, she told me simply but sternly, "Te estamos vigilando, ¿eh?" "We will be watching you." She and the others would be keeping an eye on me, not to help or protect me, but to guard against me doing anything foolish. I needed to watch my step.

Tempted to retort, "What are you implying, Norma?!" I bit my tongue and played out the line of interrogation, asking, neutrally, "What do you mean?"

She didn't miss a beat. Clearly this intervention had been planned for a while. "If anything happens that shouldn't while Michelle is away, we're going to notice, and she's going to find out as soon as she returns. You just need to watch yourself, Mateo. Of course, I am really going to be watching the women. I know you can't help yourselves." Right there Norma was announcing the bottom line: men cannot help themselves, so women must find ways to manage them.

It was not the first time, nor the last, that I would be told men couldn't resist the offer of sex. Norma's warning came from deep-seated concerns, and I had no doubt she meant what she said. Her mother, Ángela, had taught me a favorite expression that ran along the same lines: "¿A quién le dan pan que llore?" (Who cries when they're given bread?) It was a bit of wisdom that spoke as much to rural poverty, where you eat anything that's offered to you, as it did to men's "natural" proclivity to accept every sexual favor proffered.

Norma may have been teasing a little, but how much of her warning was just for laughs? To what extent did Norma think I was tempted to fool around in Michelle's absence? Would Norma have said the same thing to any man whose wife was gone for a couple of weeks? I didn't think she was making threats to women whose husbands left on trips. There was one notorious neighbor whose husband was a migrant worker in the United States and able to return for only a month or so every year. Over the years this woman had taken a parade of lovers after her husband left for the next eleven months. Maybe Norma planned to go on alert against that woman in case she tried to ensnare me.

What is often left out of this kind of thinking is that there is no such thing as a human body outside of time and space. Biological transformations occur throughout the life of every body, even male bodies, and these changes might even be heritable. Masculinity is not biological, but even if it were, we are not the amalgamation of two parts (biology and culture), but instead one complex whole.

The implications for understanding men's sexuality and violence is related to the idea that our minds and thoughts are separate from our physical bodies, a concept that has dominated highbrow and everyday discourse for centuries in the West. It has special resonance when it comes to male bodies. That's why we get the expression "He thinks with his dick." An equivalent for women—"She thinks with her pussy"—makes no sense in ordinary speech. That statement doesn't exist because of underlying popular attitudes about differences in what motivates and explains the sexualities of men and women—although certainly the notion that "it must be her time of month again" is prevalent, and it's analogous in pathologizing female behavior. The difference is that while women's reproductive capacity is invoked by reference to menstruation, in the case of men the implication is that they are largely motivated by their sexual urges, and more comprehensible if you imagine penises as divining rods.

Being a biological (not just a cultural) man, a father, and a husband have been central to my anthropological research: not only have I been threatened with exposure if I were caught having any *aventuras* with women not my wife, but I have been propositioned because "men gotta have it"; I have also been treated as an inferior parent because I was a man, and unduly celebrated when I defied expectations. An assumed— if usually undefined and immutable—maleness about me has always influenced how I have been treated by women as well as by other men. My sexuality as a man has succumbed to a taken-for-granted fetishization that is then in circular fashion attributed to my maleness itself.

Insisting on the biological roots of especially men's aberrant behavior is commonplace. Consider the following news items from the *New*

York Times on the hot-button issue of how to explain the mass murders that have become so prevalent in the contemporary United States.

From December 24, 2012

"In a move likely to renew a longstanding ethical controversy, geneticists are quietly making plans to study the DNA of Adam Lanza, 20, who killed 20 children and seven adults in Newtown, Conn. [on December 14, 2012]. Their work will be an effort to discover biological clues to extreme violence." The researchers from the University of Connecticut quickly responded to the massacre and were going to look for genetic mutations associated with mental illness, or those that might have made Lanza more prone to violence.[4]

From October 26, 2017

"Las Vegas Gunman's Brain Will Be Scrutinized for Clues to the Killing," the headline boasted. The content of the article was more modest. Dr. Hannes Vogel, director of neuropathology at Stanford University Medical Center, was going to examine the brain of the man who earlier that month had killed fifty-eight concertgoers. "The magnitude of this tragedy has so many people wondering how it could have evolved," the pathologist offered, quickly adding that he doubted he would find anything. Rather, "all these speculations out there will be put to rest, I think."[5]

What if these scientists did find some brain abnormalities? What could be the possible ramifications here? Find a gene for the perpetrators behind most mass killings in the United States—young, male, white people? And then what? Mass testing of DNA of all white males under a certain age who live in the United States? Prevalent attitudes about whiteness (as well as masculinity and youth) take for granted that their sociodemographic status is not the key to understanding their actions. Imagine if most mass murderers were young African American males. We would never hear the end racial profiling pertaining to the backgrounds, families, and personalities of these young men. Why no racial and gender profiling when it's white male youths?

The popular perception that brain disease, mental disorder, and aberrant psychological states alone could trigger mass murders in Newtown in 2012, Columbine in 1999, Oklahoma City in 1995, and Las Vegas in 2017, to mention only a few examples, may seem compelling to many, but it misses key factors. So does simply noting that 42 percent of the guns in the world are in the hands of people in the United States. Gun ownership is related to mass killings, but it does not in itself explain them. To be sure, in the United States in 2017 there were around 101 guns for every 100 residents (the highest ratio in the world). But this does not explain not just why there are fewer mass murders in Saudi Arabia (where there are 35 guns per 100 residents), Finland (34 per 100), Uruguay (32 per 100), and France (31 per 100), but why there is such a negligible number of them in those places. And although gun ownership in Switzerland is not, as is sometimes said, compulsory, the Swiss do maintain what can fairly be called an active "gun culture," focused on hunting, that has never spilled over into mass shootings.[6]

Even if we find biological indicators of troubled minds, or when we note the astronomical number of guns owned by people in the United States compared to most of the rest of the world, that still doesn't explain why mental illness among young white men manifests in the United States more than anywhere else in the form of collective killings. Nor does turning up oddities in the brain tell us anything automatically about behavior. No one could argue that genetic anomalies found in the brains of mass killers in the United States are unique to those with US birth certificates. Yet mass killings are far, far more common in the United States than anywhere else on earth outside of war zones. Why aren't masculinity, youth, and whiteness seen as key social factors in every news story, police report, and postmortem review? That is perhaps the most troubling question: Why are mass murderers typically young white men from the United States?[7]

Perhaps we should be more open-minded about those seeking the biological origins of mass murders. Maybe they'll turn something up, and at worst they will be wasting only their own time. But it is not just a matter of being open to the possibility of root biological explanations to explain social trauma such as mass killings. The danger lies in thinking we can resolve social problems through biological diagnoses any more than we can understand and resolve social inequalities through biological reasoning. The history of racial profiling on IQ in the United States should help us appreciate the alarming consequences of relying on this framework to solve questions of motive and prevention in mass murders. Yet we continue to look to biology for more answers than it can provide.

This problem of tracing men's bad behavior to genetics and hormones is getting more pronounced and pernicious, including in the general pathologization of violence as deviant and a product of the "criminally insane." Just as sanity shows itself in untold ways, so, too, insanity. Crazy doesn't in itself cause violence or war. If mass murderers didn't find receptive audiences, they could end up as isolated voices yapping at shadows. At the core of mass murders in the United States are social relations anchored to whiteness, masculinity, and youth.

When people today in Shanghai, Mexico City, or Providence, Rhode Island, say that male violence is "genetic" or "innate" or "evolutionary," they are sharing a belief that in a meaningful sense people will do what they do regardless of public policy interventions, and suggesting that we could stop wasting precious resources if we stopped trying to change behavior that is inevitable, especially when this behavior reflects something so elementary as natural selection. Like it or not, the acquiescent reasoning goes, we first have to accept that often men are just acting the way they are meant to.

If blind faith in biology is advanced to explain social problems associated with men and violence, it is not mainly because science today has become too compelling to ignore: it is because social analysis of men and violence has become too anemic and unconvincing.

THE MALE BODY AS FETISH

What the history books will say in a hundred years about our compulsive itch for biobabble in 2019 is not clear. Why so many sensible denizens of earth have yielded in our time to the numbing influence of extreme forms of biological understandings when describing gender differences and relationships itself needs to be explained. Gender confusion has led to a revival of blind faith in folk biology. For many gender-conforming people, as well as more than a few nonconformers, gender and sexuality have become petrified and unbending concepts. Even within the trans-gender community, it's hard to dodge naturalized categorization.

The term often used in the United States to speak critically about the degradation of female bodies is "objectification." Women are judged by how well they conform to stereotypical standards of beauty. Undoubtedly there are examples in which men are treated in a similar fashion, but more often than with women, the male body is fetishized as an object of potency and power. Regardless of the various and antag-onistic psychoanalytic readings of fetishism (centered on the penis or its lack), the male body as cultural fetish goes a long way to explaining how maleness is simultaneously a bane and a blessing in societies in which the body and the mind are popularly considered to be distinct entities.

Consider, for example, the classic anthropological analysis: fetishes are objects with human qualities fashioned by humans. What is special about these objects is that they in turn seem to have power over the same humans who created them. This is precisely what happens so of-ten when male sexuality and aggression become fetishes: these qualities are fashioned by humans in particular cultural and historical moments but are said to have magical, deeply spiritual, properties, and then these male sexuality and aggression fetishes, almost Frankenstein-like, come back to haunt their very creators as unbridled, overpowering male impulses. Some fetishes take on animal characteristics, like guardian spirits. At the least, even if you don't fully accept them, you'd best show proper deference toward these fetishes.[8]

Examples of the fetishization of male sexuality are all around us, from beliefs regarding male adolescent masturbation to men's extramarital affairs, from men shirking responsibility in contraception to men's sex overdrives, and to men's handicapped status as engaged fathers. Yet how much are Viagra, Cialis, and Levitra about allowing men to get back their erections for sexual satisfaction, and how much are those erections tied to proving they (still, with help) have what it takes to be real men? After all, the erect penis, in humans and many other species, is the observable *ne plus ultra* when it comes to unambiguously demonstrating sexual interest and desire.

Part of the issue surrounding the treatment of male sexuality as a fetish, a supernatural force of its own, is that it represents a deeper Western philosophical tradition that separates minds and bodies. Whether the mind and body are seen as "autonomous," "corresponding," "in parallel," or in some other arrangement, and even if they are appreciated as separate but equal, the idea that minds and bodies (in this case, male) act in some way separately "on their own" feeds too easily into attributing more automatic responses in the actions of men, and in that way to acquiescence to male bad behavior. When we look at the brains of mass murderers and ask, "What went wrong?," if we don't ignore the fact that virtually all mass murderers are men, but simply view this as a biological clue to such an extreme form of aggression, we miss the social clues that might or might not be related to some distinct morphology present in their bodies, and how cultural norms of aggression may have activated changes in body chemistry and composition.

Anthropologists use the term "ascribed" to mean what you're born with and compare this with "acquired," meaning what you learn along the way. If we think that the causes of mass murder are really more biological than cultural, then it will be far easier to focus on nature (vs.

nurture), bodies (vs. minds), and ascribed (vs. acquired). This whole way of framing things is problematic. As the feminist historian of science Evelyn Fox Keller put it, we need to accept that we are talking about "the mirage of space between nature and nurture"—human behavior cannot be usefully separated into such arbitrary categories, but still we imagine a space that does not exist. And, again, we need to pay close attention to the panhuman experience when it comes to men's sexuality and aggression: variation, variation, variation.[9]

Human biology does not float free of human social relationships. Consider one recent controversial example, the "gay gene." Much of the motivation of researchers who sought and then declared they had discovered the gay gene was to prove that gayness was "natural," and therefore not a matter of individual or social choice, and for those of a certain religious bent, presumably something that was God-given and God-sanctioned. Difficulties in discussing the gay gene, however, quickly emerged. What does "gay" really mean? It is so open to interpretation as to render moot a biological description, much less a biological source. All men who have sex with other men are gay, say some. Others respond that gayness is an identity, not an act. Some say it depends on who does what to whom.[10]

The problem with talking about the gay gene is, ultimately, that there is no biological material that is shared by all gay men because there is no universally accepted meaning of *gay* to begin with. The quest for the gay gene is a classic case of fetishizing the body and looking for bodily explanations (genes) to explain cultural categories (gayness).

As with male sexuality, fetishized phrases, such as "the biological or cultural roots of male violence," get us nowhere because they treat biology and culture as if they exist in hermetically sealed form. We need to focus our attention on the complex interactions that constitute male sexuality and violence, those that happen not simply on the scale of genes and the endocrinology of individuals, but on whole social bodies in particular times and places.

ASIAN APPROACHES: THE BODY INDIVISIBLE

In the contemporary United States, for most people most of the time, there is only one systematic way to approach medicine, illness, and healing, and that is through biomedicine as taught in all accredited medical schools and practiced by the approximately 1 million doctors in the country. In China, biomedicine is one of two systems of medicine: the other is called Traditional Chinese Medicine (TCM). And despite its name, "traditional," and its ancient roots, TCM is considered in China to be every bit as up to date as biomedicine among a wide range of people. Although many in the United States have heard of acupuncture, and many know it as a Chinese form of healing, and may have even experimented with it, acupuncture is widely regarded in the United States as an old-fashioned therapy. Advocates for TCM in China would view that appraisal as quaint, because for them the heart of the difference between the two medical approaches rests on the emphasis on holism and balance in TCM and the emphasis in biomedicine on separate body parts and distinct (immune, digestive, cardiovascular) systems. We can learn about changing men and male bodies by comparing TCM and biomedical practices—for example, by looking at issues like libido, how medical conditions like impotence are diagnosed, and what remedies are suggested to resolve them.[11]

The efficacy of one medical model or another is of less concern here than what we can learn from TCM to help us think about issues of male sexuality and violence. Central to its holistic approach, TCM is not based on anatomy, much less on what its practitioners regard as an artificial separation distinguishing "mind" from "body." Though to Western biomedical ears TCM might sound more mystical and quasi-religious than rooted in the physical chemical and biological world, TCM doctors tend not to cede the ground of science, and in fact, according to anthropologist Judith Farquhar, "to an increasing extent through the 1980s and 1990s, Chinese medical researchers and clinicians staked their careers on the essential scientificness of Chinese medicine." TCM doctors emphasize the unity of bodies, not their compartmentalization.[12]

The specific ramifications of TCM for men and maleness reside in the fact that "the divide between social gender and natural sex that informs our [Western] careful sex-gender distinction is not particularly pertinent to common usage in modern Chinese," writes Farquhar. Despite whatever you may think about *yin* and *yang*, for those who follow TCM the binary approach to women and men is inadequate, as is the notion that sex equals biology and gender equals social and cultural factors. What this means is that biology and culture are said to be joined in the body in irreducible ways, an approach that guides diagnoses and therapies by those practicing TCM.

In a comprehensive study of what he calls "the impotence epidemic" in China, anthropologist Everett Zhang argues that the growing reports of erectile dysfunction (ED) in China were a positive development because they reflected a rejection of the sexually repressed days of Maoist China. Now men can attend to this problem when it occurs, and they can do so without shame, because they live at a time when sexuality is recognized as a potentially healthy part of life for men and women.

In Zhang's study we learn about differences between TCM and biomedicine at every stage of a patient's care. Biomedical doctors in China tend to approach the issue of ED as one of erections, ejaculations, and above all, blood flow. TCM doctors are far more likely to note symptoms like a white coating on a man's tongue and a weak pulse, symptomatic not only of ED issues but also, more profoundly, of problems with the kidneys. They believe that blood flow is involved, but they do not identify the problem so narrowly or recommend treatment that addresses blood flow alone. Thus, biomedical urologists stress blood dynamics and the need to increase the flow of blood into the penis, while TCM practitioners most often seek to "smooth out the liver," which entails especially getting a man's *qi* (his "vital energy") to circulate along the liver meridian. This approach is said to facilitate the flow of blood to all parts of the man's body.

As one biomedical doctor also sympathetic to TCM counseled, "Chinese medicine produces better effects in terms of improving sexual desire and controlling ejaculation. It also improves the general status of the body, whereas Viagra can improve the rigidity and the frequency of erections." For TCM specialists, it is also not a matter of just substituting one newer pharmaceutical product, like Cialis, for another, older one, like red ginseng. Instead, it's a matter of addressing overall bodily issues that may seem to biomedical doctors to be unrelated to ED, or indeed, to other aspects of sexual dysfunction, or even sexuality in general. Zhang hails in particular those men who, rather than going from one system of treatment to another, circulate back and forth between them.[13]

In this way, Traditional Chinese Medicine, when applied to men's sexual problems, is presented as a new-old integrated approach to male minds and bodies. A greater awareness of the tenets of TCM by those now more captivated by biomedicine alone could move the needle away from excessive worries about male hydraulics, which are tied to engrained models of mechanical functioning in bodies in general. The interactions between blood and other bodily processes also holds the door open in TCM to not just curing what might ail men with their erections, but changing their very biologies in the course of treatment, so that erections become a mere byproduct of overall healing. When ED is identified as a problem of aging, for instance, biomedical doctors often assume that treatment through medications must continue forever. For TCM doctors, in contrast, treatment for these and other ailments can change male bodies, meaning that, at some point, treatment may no longer be necessary, as is more typically expected in the case of psychological afflictions not seen as necessarily permanent.

INHERITING REVOLUTIONARY VIOLENCE

How much men inherit the bodies they are born with, how much they are a product of their ancestors, and how much they can change about them are of course topics of popular debate all over the world. For most people, it's more than a question of where you get your curls or big feet: it can also involve a legacy of temperament. When my daughter Liliana would get fussy in Mexico City, a neighbor liked to rib me, saying she was acting "Matt-ish." For most of us, inheriting physical and personality traits from our families is most often a matter of what we have picked up from our parents. But in Mexico City one time I came across a belief that family endowments could be traced back much further. I was told about an inner warrior quality that had traveled down generations, hidden inside a family's genepool.

I learned about it all one day when I was talking with an old friend from the Santo Domingo barrio. She told me about a gender predicament that neighbors were confronting, one they had solved using similar hereditarian logic. It seemed that a young man had been getting into trouble by hanging around with a street gang. He'd gotten into real fights for the first time in his life. His parents were panicked. They knew it wasn't just something boys do. His best friend from childhood wasn't aggressive. So then, why him? They considered all the possibilities they could think of: It was not his family, because he came from a good, stable, loving home. It wasn't school, because he was doing pretty well there. Nor was it the neighborhood, because the street where they lived was usually tranquil.

Then his mother remembered something having to do with family, but three generations earlier. Her son's great-grandfather had participated in the Mexican Revolution of the 1910s, an incredibly violent time. Millions died. The great-grandfather had no doubt witnessed, and maybe participated in, all that slaughter. And he probably had passed down that manly violence in his blood to his own great-grandson. The fact that the young man didn't know about his great-grandfather seemed to prove the point even better: he couldn't be consciously mimicking ways he might imagine his great-grandfather had acted a century earlier; it had to be hereditary.

A family in anguish about a young man's violence has everything to do with gender confusion. They found relief from their distress by concluding that it started with an inherited trait, a biological craving inside the young man. Then they knew better what they were up against, and their despair could be eased. Despair and distress leads to a search for solutions. And biological solutions can be awfully attractive to those in distress.[14]

PARDON MY LAMARCK

In this time of widespread gender confusion and contestation, what we think of men as biological animals will be an important part of how much we think we can change and how much we do change. Recent work in biology holds some promise to help us realize new understandings about men's "animality," and in general this work can help ease us away from the nature-or-culture dichotomy related to men and maleness. We cannot choose to alter our DNA, but we can choose how to react to our environment, and that is our saving grace. The burgeoning field of epigenetics, however, points to significant changes in gene expression that can be *triggered* by behavior. Whether in jest or not, the words we use matter. "You're such a guy!" and "I have my manly needs!" is language that reflects ideas about men and masculinity that can be especially problematic because it belittles how malleable men actually are. Male bodies, just as much as female bodies, are more reactive and dynamic than passive and static.[15]

Since roughly 2000, the French naturalist Jean-Baptiste Lamarck (1744–1829) has been making a comeback of sorts in the new biological field known as epigenetics. Epigenetics has opened up vast new avenues of research that reassert "environmental" factors in gene expression, and some believe that changes in gene expression—and how genes are regulated differently in different environmental circumstances—might mean that the behavior of one generation can be passed on to the next.

Regardless of whether it turns out to be accurate to say that the environment, defined broadly, can change individual bodies, or that these changes can be inherited, epigenetics has already reached relevant findings with implications for changing male bodies, changing male behavior, and changing beliefs about maleness. Even at this early stage, conclusions from epigenetics research make clear that although you may not pass down the violent tendencies you used in the Mexican Revolution to your grandchildren, the interactions between genes and your surroundings matter: particular genes get more or less activated, and more or less relevant to human behavior, depending on everything from climate to war, from compassion to toxic masculinity.

What is more, even how men talk about themselves and think about themselves as men can have an impact on gene expression and in that way affect how DNA counts in men's lives. Take the question of inheritance again. Until fairly recently, "vertical" transmission of DNA from parent to offspring was how we understood genes being passed from one organism to another. Now, within the field of "horizontal gene transfer" (HGT), we are finding new evolutionary pathways. The main way that antibiotic resistance, for example, is spread is laterally. This can happen when a mobile and resistant segment of DNA gets inserted laterally into another chromosome. As with new work on epigenetics, the likelihood that HGT research will show that genetic material moves horizontally in other ways between humans opens up the possibility of relevant new insights into human behavior and relationships.

"The world is more Lamarckian than we used to be," primatologist Sarah Hrdy told me in 2014. She obviously didn't mean that the biological world was different, but that new understandings of the world had changed our obligation to Lamarck for his insights, which he offered over two centuries ago, and which had been cited ever since mainly as the butt of ridicule. Lamarck made two major claims: one was that if certain body parts were used more or less, this could have an effect on those same body parts in subsequent generations; the other was that characteristics acquired by one generation could be passed down to subsequent generations. It is this second contention that is more relevant to the field of epigenetics today. Lamarck believed, in other words, that changes in the environment could change one's physiology, and that these changes could be inherited by one's offspring.

Hrdy expanded: "Social scientists are so excited that everything is epigenetics now. Because it gets them out of a bind. They were increasingly in a bind because they were sort of being pinned with a label of claiming, 'Genes don't matter!'" Genes of course do matter, but epigenetics shows that just saying "genes matter" doesn't really tell us anything yet, because genes by themselves don't cause anything to happen, and genes themselves are not impervious to social, behavioral, and other conditional factors. Hrdy anticipated that with epigenetics it had become increasingly clear that environmental factors can change how genes are activated and come into play, and that was why social scientists would now feel a certain vindication for their perpetual insistence that factors such as social inequalities can reshape human bodies in ways that biologists only a generation earlier may have been more prone to resist in their theorizing about evolution and heredity.

If this were a true finding of epigenetics in general, then it would have direct ramifications for men and masculinity, because gender relations of inequality would involve those who are in superior, patriarchal conditions as well as those who are not, and men's bodies might get reshaped in the process just as much as women's.

Has it turned out that my friends in Mexico City were correct when they linked the violent inheritance from a peasant farmer who had participated in the Mexican Revolution to his great-grandson? Or that husbands who beat their wives can pass genes activated for violence on to their sons? Or that people who grow up in a society in which there has not been a generation without war in nearly a hundred years (such as the United States) somehow genetically absorb the violence of their progenitors? All these conclusions would be possible only if you link social and interpersonal violence with genetics from the start. Just because epigenetics may point to social factors as triggering gene expression does not mean that every social phenomenon has a gene to trigger. The rate of mass murders does not rise and fall because of misfiring neurons or testosterone overdoses or brain tumors or misactivated genes.

Many social scientists who study social problems pay little attention to biological factors; usually we treat them as background vapors. Though in certain subfields, such as medical anthropology and environmental anthropology, belittling the biological has been less prevalent, the greatest work in these subfields in recent decades has persuasively debunked claims of universal and uniform biologies, unveiling, for example, the varieties of ways to experience menopause; or disputed a narrow molecular focus on disease etiology—for example, in afflictions such as schizophrenia; and in general revealed the social roots of what biomedical practitioners more commonly diagnose as individual pathologies, in conditions, for instance, like PTSD.

As leading researchers who study the social consequences of epigenetics insist, however, studies focusing on nature and biological evolution have too often been divorced from those on nurture and social, economic, political, and cultural contexts. In a series of publications on epigenetics and Alzheimer's disease, medical anthropologist Margaret Lock makes clear that there is a renewed recognition among some scientists of "a molecularized 'social body' situated in time and space." According to Lock, "This shift in epigenetics is not so much away from genetics and genomics as it is moving beyond them as the new science explicitly demotes the reductive agency of genes." Lock's further challenge is for social scientists to consider "the social ramifications of this shift."[16]

As much as epigenetics has vindicated social scientists' beliefs in sociocultural and economic factors in determining human behavior, it has helped even more to provide biologists a way out, a framework within which to examine interactions between genes and environment, and an escape route from the straitjacket of biological provincialism. However, scientists have only begun to scratch the surface of what epigenetics might imply for men and maleness, including the socially contingent nature of pernicious forms of masculinity. Renegotiating and reshaping masculinity depend on a fuller appreciation of not only the pervasiveness of certain kinds of male behavior but, especially today, their conditional and unfixed potential.

Yet to talk of environmental factors is not yet to emerge from another kind of provincialism, that which makes the unit of analysis the individual or family. The full significance of epigenetics will be shackled if left there; political and economic circumstances, such as poverty, racism, and patriarchy, must be factored in. Indeed, it is in such comprehensive considerations, in integrating nature and nurture, genes and their social activation, that epigenetics can also resonate most with the fundamentals of Traditional Chinese Medicine, in particular the objective of unifying more strictly biomedical aspects and more properly social elements into a holistic description of the individual body, the social body, and even the body politic.[17]

Caution is required here. We should not yet jump to the conclusion that our lifestyle alters our genes and that we will pass these changes on to our children. As Lock and coauthor Gisli Palsson write, "whether or not epigenetic changes are transmitted intergenerationally in humans remains a matter for heated debate, but [even] if this proves not to be the case, irrefutable evidence shows that epigenetic changes arise anew in ensuing generations if living conditions are not substantially improved." They conclude, "A major perceptual shift is underway; one in which the gene has been demoted and nature/nurture is conceptualized as an *indivisible* entity, albeit malleable, in which nurture is the active, initiating force, to which the genome reacts."[18]

One potentially important lesson from the first decades of epigenetics research is surely that, as with "male hormones" (aka testosterone), men's Y chromosomes have been getting a bad rap, or at least they have had to bear more than their fair share of the blame for folk biology addressing men, maleness, and violence. Men's sexual assaults on women (and other men) are no more genetically driven or governed—and male aggressors no more deserving of impunity—than poor communication skills are the leading cause of military invasions and occupations. Biology has been used in recent decades to provide inscrutable evidence about why men's indiscretions (and worse) seem so widespread and deep-seated, along with the implication that we can physically restrict men, but cannot really hope to physically change them. We need to be skeptical about these pervasive and malignant beliefs. Bioskepticism is not a dismissal of biology. Instead it calls our attention to the need to make chromosomes, anatomy, and evolution far more scrutable and accountable to all.

In a paper on the new science of epigenetics, historian of science Sarah Richardson concludes "that epigenetics may counter traditional ideological conceptions of male and female differences by documenting a diversity of sexual phenotypes and that epigenetics may provide methods for studying the biological embodiment of gender by yielding mechanisms for the environmental and social mediation of sex." Among other things, bioskepticism will help us get out of the business of conducting biopsies on the brains of mass murderers only to discover they are young, white, American males. That evidence was available to us before we began picking apart their brains. The significance of epigenetics for men and masculinities is not simply that maleness is not preordained, or that talk to the contrary is bad science, but that denying the interactions between environment and human biology is harmful to men's social recovery and revitalization.[19]

CHAPTER TEN

DON'T LET MEN OFF THE HOOK

Unaccommodated man is no more
but such a poor, bare, forked animal as thou art.

Lear to Edgar and Fool, *King Lear*,
WILLIAM SHAKESPEARE

EFORE WE CAN UNYOKE MALENESS FROM MANLINESS, BEFORE WE
can reexamine social policies based on faulty beliefs about virile
compulsions, we need to abandon much of our biological language
about men and masculinity. Human sex is not best understood as a form
of animal mating. War is not explicable by blood tests for paternity, testosterone levels, or anything else that relates to men's physiologies. Any
science, new or old, that is used to legitimate and maintain unequal
social relations, if it is repeated often enough, can take on the veneer of
inevitability over time. Questionable science gets normalized into a fog
of half-baked but influential ideas. This is a time of gender confusion
with the potential for gender renegotiations. It is unlikely women who
have gained access to positions denied their grandmothers will cede
ground, but there is no doubt that there are conservative forces that
would like them to do just that.

Reshaping modern masculinity affects men and the women with whom men share their lives. We have nothing to fear from biology, but only from folk biology that lets men off the hook and sells men short. We are at a crossroads in thinking about modern masculinities around the world, and we must come to terms with the biological determinants of men and maleness. How should men act? Treat others? What can be changed about men and masculinities? Biology should mean opportunity, not destiny.

We need to know why only men are subject to military conscription, why there is no modern form of contraception for men, why men still dominate in government, business, and cultural life in every country on earth. Are these social facts inevitable, or are they not? Recent decades have brought enormous changes in the power of women in every facet of social life, so perhaps the answer is too obvious. But these changes have also brought renewed confusion and challenge to fundamental ideas about gender. And the backlash is formidable. One distressingly popular author writes in his rules for life of the quest for vindication on behalf of all men who feel left out of these developments empowering women. For "every spurned male" who feels denigrated by talk of gender equality, Jordan Peterson appears to counsel that revenge is the reasonable antidote to the chaos that he says has intensified as a result of women's assertiveness.[1]

We need to know why men rape. Is it primarily a matter of natural male responses to stimuli? Talk about rape culture on college campuses and throughout society predated the #MeToo movement of the late 2010s. But it picked up momentum as women and men debated the degree to which rape is something all men are capable of committing, whether more men would rape if they thought they would not be caught and punished, how much rape was cultural, and how much it was natural to the male biology and essence. These discussions are vital if we are to address the problem of sexual assault, and they are opportunities that can help us clarify our language and our beliefs about men, maleness, aggression, and sexuality.

We need to know why racialized ideas about biological capacities and animal impulses are, in the main, publicly marginal and despised in the academy and mainstream media—although they become more dangerous in periods of white supremacist resurgence—but beliefs about men's biological capacities and animal urges have them as barely removed from the state of feral beasts. Turn on any news program, read any account of gender issues, and you will invariably hear about testosterone, Y chromosomes, alpha males, and boys who will be boys. Reducing certain kinds of people to animals has historically been an effective way to pigeonhole them. Animals are incapable of reason, they must be controlled, and they should not be allowed to make decisions for themselves or others. If you doubt the existence of a widespread belief that men are in some fundamental sense not able to control themselves because they are men, the way a shark cannot help eating a seal, then think instead about alpha gorillas, and about how often their sexual predations and aggressive behaviors are compared to the behaviors of human males. A guy's gotta do what a guy's gotta do. Admittedly, this is infinitely more complex because men are in control of so many aspects of our social, economic, and political life; still, and crucially, we gain absolutely nothing if we believe that men, because they are male, are obliged by nature to act in preordained ways, good or bad.

Language can shift perceptions. And narrow-minded ideas about men and maleness employing scientific jargon can be contested. For one thing, we can expand our understanding of what it means to be a male animal. For another, we can learn to use a less extreme vocabulary to describe the actual experiences of people born with bodies that supposedly confer one or another identity on them. The greatest problem arises when we accommodate men because we believe that they are at their core animals who cannot help themselves, and when we come to believe that we cannot change that fact of life, evolution, and DNA. That, like it or not, men can at best be constrained from their irrepressible compulsions.[2]

THEY/THEM/THEIRS

If the term "gender binary" sounds like jargon, that's because you haven't been around students lately. "Male" and "female" no longer work for everyone as the only possible categories. For today's college students, the clear line dividing male from female often looks a lot fuzzier than it did to past generations. Like with the words "discourse" and "plutocracy," all it takes is a political movement to move a word from the academic lingo column to the list of popular phrases. Generation Z, born between the mid-1990s and the mid-aughts, is at the forefront of this movement. One of the ways they are challenging the gender binary is by shedding the pronouns they were raised with and adopting "they" to replace "he" and "she."

The pronoun moment might be a movement akin to their mothers' demand for a shift from Mrs. and Miss to Ms. And like the title shifts of that earlier generation, today the They Movement is part of widespread and intense discussions on college campuses in the United States about larger issues, in this case about queerness, gayness, and transgender politics. How influential they will be in the long run remains to be seen, but their rejection of the gender binary certainly holds important insights and lessons about gender confusion, the science of maleness, and thinking rooted in the detection of gonads to understand basic issues of gender identity.[3]

When introducing themselves at the first meeting of a club or campus organization, students at Brown University often include a new factoid. In addition to name, year, and major, they give their preferred pronouns: *he/him/his, she/her/hers*, or *they/them/theirs*, or something else entirely. In a remarkably quick adoption of new gender norms that began in the mid-2010s, it has since become routine in casual conversations as well as classrooms. In response, younger faculty began asking for pronoun information on the first day of classes, and many students are putting their preferred pronouns on their email signatures. In just a few years, students have campaigned for greater acceptance of gender and sexual fluidity, trying to move beyond the neat gender frames of their parents and grandparents. Sometimes these issues are tied to queerness, but not always. Sexual orientation is often treated as a separate, if related, set of issues.

Students are challenging either-or restrictions and dichotomous ways of dividing up the world between two neat groups of men and women. But the United States is not the only place where these dichotomies have prevailed. The fact is that most cultures throughout history have categorized people into male and female. Anthropologists studying New Guinea talk of sexual and gender "polarity" as not just pervasive there but universal, even considering the male initiation rituals practiced among the Sambia and others described in Chapter 1. In a mean-spirited defense of the gender binary, Prime Minister Edouard Philippe of France declared in 2017 that he was banning the use of gender-neutral language in government documents. For my students, however, the demand to "break down the binary!" is an urgent and righteous objective. Youths around the world today are so dissatisfied with the strict male-female classification system that they are championing new ways of cataloging gender.[4]

One of my students told me about an invitation he had received: "Hey guys, I just wanted to throw a party to celebrate the 2 year anniversary since I started hormones and all the wonderful things that happened after that. Let's celebrate spring and femininity in whatever form that means for you!" They called it the Hormone Party to raise money for their friend, who was transitioning. In recent years, trans people have challenged the idea that gender identity is sacrosanct, often contesting this view with a far more wide-ranging commitment to gender justice and social justice in general. When they are treated as "impossible people who are not who we say we are, cannot exist, cannot be classified, and cannot fit anywhere," this is a denial of the slipperiness of gender identity categories and a negation of gender diversity and inclusion. The emergence of trans social movements that refuse to get shoehorned into now more acceptable categories of gay and lesbian is an affront to social mores in a society already having a hard time coping with what it means to be a man or a woman. Transpolitics expand a distrust of whatever has been called normal, perhaps as part of a search for what French philosopher Michel Foucault called "the happy limbo of non-identity."[5]

All told, there is great variation in how trans people live gender and sex. For some it is a binary affair, and transitions seek to bring union to body and mind. For others, a primary goal in life is to escape such dualisms altogether. When Caitlyn Jenner appears on the front cover of *Vanity Fair*, it is not as an ambiguously gendered person. And there lies the rub: when bodies are realigned with identities, as radical as it all might seem, there can appear to be only two gendered possibilities, and trans experiences are used to demonstrate this. The gender binary is a powerful whirlpool that can pull down even the unruliest gender insurgents into its vortex. As trans scholar Jack Halberstam has written, "the concept of being without a gender, however, is whimsical at best, since there are few ways to interact with other human beings without being identified with some kind of gendered embodiment." When strictly dichotomous thinking about gender begins to fray at the edges and impede new ideas, authorities on all things male and female either begin to question foundational premises or their work ossifies. We are too prone to casual, unthinking, and harmful stereotypes about male sexuality.[6]

Calling yourself queer in college today can be an act of solidarity as well as an announcement of sexual interests. A student from Mexico describes his friends who have come out as gay as also having become "queer over time." In a series of studies of cowboys in northern Mexico who are married to women and call themselves straight, but who nonetheless regularly have sex with other men, anthropologist Guillermo Núñez-Noriega describes how identity and behavior may sometimes seem at odds. Or, better put, how they can seem at odds to those who lack the imagination to envision gender, sex, and sexuality in any language other than what they are used to. For some of my students who don't identify as queer, these Mexican *vaquero*-cowboys, reminiscent of characters in the movie *Brokeback Mountain*, defy their basic views about men and masculinity and suggest gender-nonconforming options. A queer lens helps them to think outside a dualistic default framework, either gay or straight.[7]

Where the They Movement will go is far from clear. There are already signs it is spreading throughout society, including on television programs (Showtime's *Billions*) and in the workplace; pronoun innovations are likely to increase as today's students graduate and start jobs. But in the closing years of the 2010s, students are once again pioneering new ways of thinking and talking about being gendered persons. They are asking that we add some new ways of talking about gender that allow for the growing gender fluidity they experience in their lives. As always, the lodestar we chase is breaking with inflexible ways of understanding men and masculinity dressed up in the language of biology, and discovering the numerous ways in which maleness is being reconsidered and renegotiated in different social contexts around the world as we approach the 2020s.

If double vision is all we perceive when we look at gender, then it's time for new glasses. Any way you slice it, the gender binary looks like it is headed for phased retirement. Although our biologies have not changed in many a millennia, what it means to be a man or a woman has altered in fundamental ways over decades. Biology narrowly construed can no more explain culture than culture narrowly construed can explain biology.[8]

HIGH SCHOOL BEASTS

On October 6, 2018, by a vote of 50 to 48, the US Senate confirmed Brett Kavanaugh as associate justice of the US Supreme Court. The social schisms that troubled the nation through the outpouring of protest against and in defense of Kavanaugh revealed more than just the fact that many senators and citizens believed his denials of sexual assaults on women in high school and later, more than just that many felt that even if he did these things it should be chalked up to youth, and not held against him forever, and more than just that so many people could overlook his sexual assaults because they liked his conservative politics. Support for Kavanaugh from high and low also showed what millions of men and women wanted, or at least expected, from a man, especially a man of high accomplishment and naked ambition.

What we have here is an example of what anthropologist Tanya Luhrmann called "a moral vision that treats the body as choiceless and nonresponsible and the mind as choice-making and responsible." The Kavanaugh hearings signaled the issue by implicitly distinguishing between his responsible judicial (i.e., mental) capacity, on the one hand, and his all-too-male body, on the other, which provided fewer options for controlling his actions, especially with respect to women. The spectacle implied that when people happen to inhabit male bodies, it is futile to try to hold them truly accountable: the best we can hope to accomplish is to find effective mechanisms to contain men in their rawest form.[9]

It would be easy to limit discussion to the performances of the key actors in the infamous hearings that led to Kavanaugh's confirmation: The federal judge becomes frantic, infuriated, vengeful. He screams at Democratic senators who have the temerity to ask about his drinking habits, demanding they reveal their own. Women protesters gather in the thousands, infiltrate the hearing room, bang on doors, shout down the nominee. What Kavanaugh deems appropriate behavior—crying, taunting, and all-around belligerence—flows seamlessly with what many observers presume are lies under oath about his high school yearbook and calendar entries from that time. The key actors contend over matters juridical and political. But the heart of the confirmation deliberations revolves around gender and sexuality, the collision of fundamental convictions about what men are and what they are not, what they can be and what they cannot be, what they do and why they do it.

If you're reading this book, my censure of Kavanaugh and his supporters may be so much preaching to the choir. Yet it is too easy to sling arrows at tyrants alone. We also need to be self-critical. It is easy for all of us to downplay how we teach men to behave in certain ways, and how we spread the cultural ideas that create the illusion that men are the victims of their own biology. In that spirit, I offer relevant editorial comments regarding Kavanaugh and the hearings from two widely read liberal social observers, *New York Times* op-ed columnist Frank Bruni and philosopher Martha Nussbaum.

The Supreme Court seat hung in the balance. The issues focused on men, maleness, and male sexual violence against women, all of which were crying out for thorough and sophisticated description and analysis. In an op-ed about Brett Kavanaugh, Frank Bruni wrote, "That's him riding a wave of testosterone and booze, among similarly pumped-up, zonked-out buddies." It was a potential learning moment on all counts, an opportunity to take discussion about masculinity seriously, to introduce new insights and findings, and not simply to repeat formulaic ideas about what causes men to sexually assault women. Yet instead we were tutored again about the liability all teen boys carry in them, the scariest of all biological compounds, testosterone.[10]

What's wrong with a frivolous reference to a hormone? What's wrong with a colorful turn of phrase, given that Bruni's underlying message was a scathing rebuke of Kavanaugh? What's misguided is the unintentional but explicit suggestion that teenage boys have a chemical that makes them do things they would not otherwise do; that if you are a boy and have this chemical in abundance, then you, too, will do such things; and that the problem with Kavanaugh's sexual attacks can be meaningfully traced not to the character of the individual boy or to the specific act of sexual attack but instead to an adverse mix of testosterone and alcohol in a generic male body. Of all the things Frank Bruni could have written about Brett Kavanaugh, why testosterone? Was testosterone to blame, even in part?

What's wrong is that neither testosterone nor alcohol *makes* anyone do anything. In the case of testosterone, unless Kavanaugh had abnormally high levels of it (an assertion no one has made), the argument is untenable. If there is any correlation between violent activity and testosterone, it is that the violent activity may cause the level of the hormone to rise, not the other way around. If you are going to employ the term testosterone, you should know that and teach that. As for alcohol, it may disinhibit people and encourage their pent-up desires, but it is not causal. If you are not repressing an urge to sexually assault people, no amount of booze will oblige you to abuse another person, any more than intoxication on an airplane will in itself force you out of your seat to dance in the aisles. To hold an organic substance inside Kavanaugh's male body accountable for his actions is to legitimize egregious behavior.

By using testosterone as an explanation in this way we might as well be back with Lyndon Johnson and one of his more memorable responses when reporters asked him why the United States persisted in Vietnam: "Johnson found it difficult to sustain his rationality in dealing with war critics," according to one historian. "During a private conversation with some reporters who pressed him to explain why we were in Vietnam, Johnson lost his patience. According to Arthur Goldberg, L.B.J. unzipped his fly, drew out his substantial organ and declared, 'This is why!'" To attribute Kavanaugh's sexual assaults to testosterone in any way is to argue, in essence, that we may not like it, but, dammit, that's just the way men are, especially powerful men like Lyndon Johnson and potential Supreme Court justices. It not only exonerates men for their individual and military assaults, it tells boys and men that this is just what is anticipated from the most manly men.[11]

In an essay on the Kavanaugh hearings, Martha Nussbaum wrapped up an old trope in a new skin: "And then, beneath the hysteria," she wrote, "lurks a more primitive emotion: disgust at women's animal bodies. Human beings are probably hard-wired to find signs of their mortality and animality disgusting, and to shrink from contamination by bodily fluids and blood. . . . But in every culture male disgust targets women, as emblems of bodily nature, symbolic animals by contrast to males, almost angels with pure minds."[12]

What is most curious to me about Nussbaum's comments is that, if anything, the symbolic performance was precisely the opposite: Kavanaugh was on full bestial display, while Christine Blasey Ford, the woman who courageously accused him of the early sexual assault, was judicious and analytical in her crafted statements. Nothing in the hearings bore out Nussbaum's particular gendered representations and imaginings. Kavanaugh was a beast whose unleashed nature was completely reasonable to his supporters. The abject lesson was that if his blood boiled, this is just what happens when you corner a wild animal. (And Kavanaugh, of course, was not the only one to rage: Senator Lindsey Graham's rant during the hearings was likewise keyed to demonstrating unbridled, visceral rage and intimidation.) The debate about the teenage years bore out that adolescent boys are like unbroken stallions. Neither beatific behavior nor rational performance from Kavanaugh was in evidence, nor was either of these encouraged.

Kavanaugh's demeanor in congressional sessions was the opposite of aberrant; he was entirely in tune with the times, giving free rein to the inner male. And the same thing is happening around the world. In China, for example, the God of Biology has partially supplanted Confucius (and Mao) in providing the basis for understanding men and masculinities. My colleague Lingzhen Wang has noted that "primitive passion, raw sexuality, and natural instincts embodied by minority or rural men became vital in this articulation of postsocialist Chinese manhood." Conjectures about men and women, whether in China, in Mexico, or in the United States, are too often based on essentialized gender categories, betraying overreliance on what Stephen Jay Gould called "speculative stories" about human behavior—here, about men, maleness, and masculinity. In this way we are developing proscriptions for social policy founded on those same faulty conjectures and end up preventing clearer analysis about key issues, such as why men assault women and what we can do to stop them.[13]

As a result of feminist perseverance, we are perhaps now more cautious than in the past about using red-flag terms to describe women,

such as "hysterical," "emotional," "whiny," and "conniving." We need
to pay attention to corresponding expressions about men that are not
helpful. The more we avoid phrases that reduce women to a shared set
of impulse-responses, the more we allow women to experiment with who
they are and what they want. Unless we do the same for men, we condemn them to reacting to the world through preordained bodily pressures, with far nastier consequences for everyone else. If we call a man
brutish we might have a very specific image in mind about what kind of
person he is, or how he has acted on some occasion. The same could be
said if we call a woman bossy. But who benefits, and at what cost?

If toxic masculinity is antithetical to what a good man should be,
what exactly is the opposite of toxic masculinity? It was not hard to find
examples of famously nontoxic men on the Internet in the 2010s. People were looking for a different kind of male hero. Former pro football
players and movie stars often headed the lists of the most nontoxic masculine men; the point seemed to be that you could be a big, strong guy
and still not want to mistreat women and other men. Fair enough. Still,
we continued to operate in restricted air space: you flew as masculine or
feminine (presumably based on your equipment), and your only choice
was what kind of masculine or feminine.

The whole point of talking about toxic masculinity is, or should be,
to critique a form of noxiousness that employs masculinity to make its
point and enforce its rule. It's a good thing that the term "toxic masculinity" came into being: it's a jolting critique that captures pernicious
and harmful male behavior. Perhaps the phrase "male behavior" still
slides too easily into thinking there's something about being male, but
toxic masculinity provides us with a way to talk about particular kinds
of widespread and destructive behavior that is especially associated with
certain forms of maleness. We need this kind of language if we are to address gender inequalities. But caution is also warranted, so we don't go
digging for roots to the problem that don't exist, in this case an imagined
inherent need for men to embody good or bad kinds of masculinity.

We sometimes say certain attributes are especially manly or womanly, or we associate particular ways of interacting with gender. We may think of cooperation as feminine, for example, and of domination as masculine. But if the goal is simply to alter the trait list for what constitutes masculinity, we remain stuck in the same binary gender ruts. By buying into the idea that alternative, nontoxic masculinities should emphasize cooperation over domination, we are essentially arguing that men, because they are men, have to act in masculine ways, so let's expand the definition of what masculine can include.

Neither cooperation nor domination has to be embedded in gender, however. And really, there is no mandatory requirement for the labels "masculinity" and "femininity" in the first place. They have been central to human relationships, but they are not ultimately essential to them. They can be diverting to play with, but they can be tremendous burdens. In the end, we do not need separate trait lists for masculine and feminine any more than we do for left-handers versus right-handers. To maintain these beliefs in gendered ways only helps to perpetuate unhelpful explanations that drag us back into identifying every behavior as either masculine or feminine, a framework that only makes sense if their distinct biologies oblige men to operate within one set of parameters and women another.

THE RULE OF ALPHA MALES

Gender confusion has stirred more than a few women and men to speak out against the abuses of powerful men and their personal and social ways of domination. These voices have made clear that their distress is widespread and deep, and it has led to righteous protest throughout the world. Growing numbers of women and men have sought ways to explain, without excusing, the behavior of these men. Disentangling taken-for-granted ideas about men's natures, their bodies, and their biologies is at the heart of addressing the distress arising from gender confusion.

The extent to which popular scientific frameworks about men, maleness, and male sexuality and aggression permeate our thinking is alarming. A major 2006 World Bank document on men, masculinity, and gender in development instructs us in this way:

> The concept of alpha and beta males has come to social science from animal biology, particularly the study of primates. Consider the notion that beta males may be systematically overlooked within their social structures (or within the social structures on whose sidelines they lurk). These may include men who are homeless, alcoholic, imprisoned, mentally ill, disabled, or just plain socially inept. The image conveyed by a range of derogatory terms in English—geek, loser, nerd—is clearly that of a male.
>
> Indeed, much of the focus on gender inequality in contemporary societies comes from comparing the alpha, or "winner" males, with the situation of women."[14]

If theories of nonhuman primate categories like alpha and beta males are used by the World Bank to guide its personnel in how to distribute hundreds of millions of dollars in gender equity aid, and through this report to suggest that human male behavior is directly connected to biological and evolutionary presumptions, we're beginning from a perilous starting point. If alpha male primates have something to tell us not only about men's violence and sexuality, but about their migratory patterns, their fathering conduct, their leadership techniques, and their food preferences, life expectancy, hygienic habits, and speaking and sitting styles, then remedial efforts are crippled out of the gate. In particular, comparing human males with the males of other primates in a book about human men and masculinities requires a narrowly biologistic framework that can never fully or adequately explain individual differences among *Homo sapiens* males.

More egregiously, by associating "alpha males" across the animal kingdom as social "winners," the report's editors, Ian Bannon and Maria C.

Correia, fail to address an entire literature showing the physiological implications of being an alpha or beta male primate: one team of baboonologists, for example, reports that "alpha males exhibited much higher stress hormone levels than second-ranking (beta) males, suggesting that being at the very top may be more costly than previously thought." Stress, hypertension, suppressed immune function, mental health issues, and injuries from attempts to unseat presiding alpha males are some of the risk factors they face.[15]

Not only do the World Bank's pronouncements about men and women have major repercussions for development funding throughout the world, but they showcase the prevailing ideas about men undergirding the thinking of men (and a few women) who wield leadership power in finance, government, industry, and every other aspect of social life in every corner of the globe. It would have been one thing to slip in the phrase "alpha male"—it's hackneyed, but nothing worse than that. To evoke alpha maleness in an extended cross-species comparison trespasses into altogether more dangerous territory.

Discussing this circular reasoning to reinforce preconceptions, the anthropologist Marshall Sahlins wrote about the use and abuse of biology, including the relationship between human and nonhuman animal behavior and the reiterative history of comparative animal studies. "Since the seventeenth century," he said, "we seem to have been caught up in this vicious cycle, alternately applying the model of capitalist society to the animal kingdom, then reapplying this bourgeoisfied animal kingdom to the interpretation of human society."[16]

If we expect men to act in certain ways because they are males, and think that males of all primate species have special, circumscribed, common ways of going about in the world, then how can we resist the temptation to explain and excuse male sexual assaults (and participation in war, and much else) except by recourse to biological reasoning? Writing against claims of cross-species "rape," for instance, biologist Anne Fausto-Sterling has said that using "the word *rape* to describe animal behavior robs it of the notion of will, and when the word, so robbed, once again is applied to humans, women find their rights of consent and refusal missing. Rape becomes just one more phenomenon in the natural world, a world in which natural and scientific, rather than human, laws prevail."[17]

THE AURA OF INEVITABILITY

The women's movement of the 1960s and 1970s activated a revolution in scholarship about women, and later about men. Because anthropology is in many ways the most commodious of disciplines, covering everything from human origins to gossip to power to sex in every nook and cranny on earth, second-wave feminists looked early on to anthropologists to answer several questions:

Have men always dominated women in every society and historical period in the world, and is this therefore a human universal?

When, how, and why does male authority become characteristic of human relationships?

What significant variations on these themes could anthropologists uncover that might be chalked up to cultural particularity?

Early books by feminist anthropologists tackled cross-cultural issues like the public and private lives of women and men: Did women in some societies have more power in households than they did society-wide? Or emotions: Were women and men hardwired differently, or were the differences mainly cultural? And questions of power in general: Were men in charge everywhere and throughout history? If you could find significant exceptions to this general state of affairs, then you could prove it was not some essential and irreversible part of human social arrangements. If you couldn't, some argued, that proved something basic about evolution and inevitability.

Among the earliest and boldest of the insurgent anthropologists was Sherry Ortner. In a 1972 essay read widely by scholars and activists alike—and one that could have been the inspiration for Martha Nussbaum's 2018 Brett Kavanaugh piece—Ortner argued that "the secondary status of woman in society is one of the true universals, a pan-cultural fact." Her purpose, she stressed, went far beyond mere academics: "I wish to see genuine change come about, the emergence of a social and cultural order in which as much of the range of human potential is open to women as it is open to men."[18]

The reason women and men went along with the order of things, and had since time immemorial, she said, rested on ingrained cultural thinking that accepted women's inferior status in running the affairs of state and socially significant institutions. A few simple examples illustrate her point: in 2018, nearly five decades after Ortner wrote her essay, less than 20 percent of the 115th US Congress were women; since 1789, only 52 US senators had been women. Moreover, in 2018, only twenty-five women were CEOs of Fortune 500 companies. In Mexico, women got the vote in 1947, but only at the municipal level. It was not until 1953 that they could vote for president and stand for elections. And not until 1983 were they welcome in *cantinas*.

It would be hard to question Ortner's position that women's leadership was and still is devalued in the United States and other societies. Rwanda, which has the highest percentage of women (a majority) in its national parliament, has arrived there through stringent quotas demanded by foreign powers. To extend Ortner's analysis: it is not biology that leads to the second-class status of women in every society, but cultural prejudice, complicity, and indolence.

Yet Ortner went further, insisting not only that men were universally identified more closely than women with culture, but that women were symbolically associated more often with nature. In English, we talk about Mother Nature, not Father Nature. Beginning with women's bodies and their "natural" procreative functions, Ortner believed, women have always been tied to the reproduction of life, while men (who don't have this creative ability) need to create culturally, socially, and politically.

This men-are-to-culture as women-are-to-nature thesis generated heated debate. Entire books were published critiquing Ortner for her concept. There is no universally accepted meaning of "nature," for example, so it's hard to say women are always more associated with it: it represents different things in different contexts. Counterexamples were easy to come by. Ortner's conclusions rested on gender universals that looked increasingly problematic given the vast array of gender relationships and practices in the world and historically.[19]

Ortner developed her own response, though, in which she essentially doubled down on her original contentions but added an escape clause. In a 1996 essay, she concluded that universal male dominance was an accurate characterization, and that her symbolic association of men with culture and women with nature was correct. However, she now added, all these identities and beliefs represented, more than anything else, "an unintended consequence of social arrangements designed for other purposes."

Early divisions of labor in hunter-gatherer groups were influenced by who gets pregnant, experiences childbirth, and lactates versus who does not, with those who do not BEING presumably more available for roaming after game. It all snowballed over the millennia, with men fulfilling many functions and needs on larger and larger social scales, to a point where men directed governance and commerce everywhere and always. No one set out to do this, there was no intent on the part of men to seize power from women; but just as certainly, explanations were developed by men and women to justify and promote this gendered arrangement, and, as Ortner supposes, "men as it were lucked out."[20]

Is that all there is to it then? Does the patriarchy come down to no more than a matter of luck? To some extent, and fortunately, it does. Because the alternative explanations as to why men are in charge could be that there is something predetermined by God or by DNA. Inequality, oppression, and patriarchy are not inherent in gender divisions of labor at the level of societies any more than in families. But they can be, and there's the rub. We can all go around believing in the inevitability of men being in charge as the normal state of affairs, like it or not, defend it or not. But among the things that distinguish human animals from the other kinds is the ability to take stock of situations and change attitudes and behavior in radical directions.

And we humans can directly address certain physical factors that have contributed to this long-standing gender division of labor. For starters, although it takes parts from a man and a woman to make a woman pregnant, and women, not men, give birth and nurse—we can change several of these "facts of life." There is nothing stopping men from feeding their babies and being the primary caregivers for their children or adopting children of their own. Especially in the twentieth century, more than ever before in human and animal history, sexual reproduction became changeable in ways never before imagined. Indeed, by the end of the twenty-first century, it may become possible for men to give birth and lactate under certain circumstances (for example, with uterine transplantation or an artificial uterus, combined with hormone treatments). It is inconceivable that male chimpanzees (or bonobos, for that matter) could be taking on primary child-rearing duties in one hundred years. Maternal mortality went from a serious challenge for women worldwide as recently as 1900 to a problem for women lacking access to good health care in 2000. Although there is still a long way to go, especially among marginalized populations, reproduction and reproductive health for billions of women globally has been seriously improved over the past one hundred years—among other things, allowing for new opportunities to bridge male/female divides that we may have long assumed were inevitable, and opening up new possibilities for our understanding of gender, sex, and sexuality for people of all kinds. It's not hard to see that until fairly recently, when modern, reliable forms of birth control for human females became available, women had a lot more reason to be "choosy" about how often they had sex and with whom, and that over the centuries this choosiness could easily be mistaken for something natural in human females.

With these changes and the social and political pressures of the world of the future, gender divisions of labor could be contested as never before in human history. Indeed, they have been challenged in the twentieth and twenty-first centuries with the changes we have already seen. At this fortuitous moment in the history of scientific advances relating to human reproduction, it would be terrible, in my opinion, to hang onto outmoded ways of thinking about men and women that would otherwise interfere with the fullest possible expression of new gender identities and ways of sharing activities like child care.

Whether men have been fortunate or not to wield authority down through the ages, Ortner's analysis of men lucking out is much more satisfactory than assuming men are animalistic machines who lack women's supposedly innate and fundamental ability to nurture their offspring, much less to control their own inoperable inner impulses. As the fable goes, the elephant got its long trunk when one day a crocodile pulled on a youngster's previously much shorter nose. Ever since then, elephants have had stretched-out snouts. That's known as a just-so story. Boys will be boys because they're made that way, they will always be that way, and they can't help themselves any more than mallard ducks can around female ducks. That's another just-so story.

Beyond the fact that culture and nature mean different things to different people, and whether men have ever actually been more associated with culture (whatever that means) and women with nature (the same), today it is worth considering the extent to which this association is often the reverse in the popular imagination. To be sure, rational and scientific thought is still widely considered more masculine than feminine—and emotions more feminine than masculine. Yet without falling into the opposite overreach, we could also conclude that in crucial respects in many parts of the overly biologized world, men are now popularly linked to nature, in that their sexuality and aggression are said to originate in their barely controllable bodies. Women are widely expected to provide cultural balance to counteract men's animality, so that men can't do more social and familial harm than they would if left to their own devices.

How and when men are considered closer to nature than women today in Shanghai, Mexico City, or Providence, Rhode Island, is related in no small part to people believing in this kind of gender fatalism. Any belief system that places the males of our species beyond the pale, picturing them as powerless to change, puts one hell of a historical burden on our boys—and our girls.

Why does so much of this naturalized folk biology about men pass muster with the same people who righteously decry histories that compare nonwhite peoples to nonhuman animals, or that degrade Africans as rapacious predators, Chinese as swarming ants, and Jews as rats—and who rightly criticize the president of the United States for saying, of undocumented Mexicans, "These aren't people. These are animals." The righteousness often slips into playful jest, however, when it comes to comparisons of males in human and other species. There's just something about those men and their antics, sexual and aggressive, that seems to lend itself to spontaneous mockery. All well and good, and no doubt cathartic, when the issue is to make fun of those holding the most powerful positions in society. But when the jokes about men come to stand for comprehensive and concise analysis of them as a homogeneous category (and not just powerful men), we run the risk of living out our predictions; perhaps most importantly, we in effect tell men that although we may not approve of this or that attribute, we also understand that they in some ways can do little other than submit their corporeal selves to evolution's dictates, animal urges, lascivious impulses, and bellicose inclinations.[21]

A KICK IN THE BALLS

In the United States, the cowboy has a long and emblematic history representing a certain kind of stoic, rugged, masculine allure. The same symbol works with the Mexican *vaquero*, and in fact the folklorist Américo Paredes has traced the origins of the cult of machismo in Mexico to the

American cowboy. At one with the untamed outdoors, the cowboy image is usually completed with a horse and a magnificent, mountainous landscape in the background. The American cowboy came to be complemented by the civilizing influence of the female schoolmarm. Whatever you think nature is, cowboys might be as close as you can get to it. Schoolmarms, on the other hand, were uniquely cultured and educated. This gendered archetype has had a profound impact on the social imagination: that there are more Hollywood westerns set in the nineteenth century than there are World War I movies is testament to the prominent position of the uncivilized cowboy in society.[22]

Now I suppose there isn't anything necessarily natural about every cowboy, or inescapably cultural about every schoolmarm. But by popular consensus, these associations work. Whether popular culture provides a mirror in which we are our reflections, or images of cowboys and schoolmarms themselves plant these ideas, is something that hardly matters. Commonly shared language and representations are a vital part of making sense of the world, of relationships, of hierarchies, and of life lessons. So it may be worth noting an odd symmetry or similarity in everyday sayings in many parts of the world about a key part of the male anatomy: the testicles.

Commonplace sayings about testicles endure throughout the world, their meanings a ball of confusion. Take Mexico. If you say about someone, "El tiene muchos huevos," you are saying he has a lot of balls (literally, eggs), which means the same thing in Spanish as it does in English. But you can also say, "Es un huevón," he's ballish/eggish, indicating a man is lazy. In both cases, meaning rests on the idea that a man's testicles imbue him with his essential personal qualities, whether he is bold or lethargic. It hardly matters if you are saying something positive or negative about a man; what counts is that he has these organs and that these organs stipulate his very being and behavior.

In the same way, I am struck, and I will admit a bit disillusioned, every time I see a scene in a movie where a guy gets kicked, punched, or otherwise hit in the balls. Sure, it turns the tables when men are brought down symbolically. It's funny to see someone get their comeuppance. What bothers me is the way this happens, because each time it also says that testicles are the soul of men and masculinity, and the way to motivate a man is through his groin. It's not just in movies, of course, as boys often make a game of "goosing" each other, and men will involuntarily smile when a friend gets struck too hard in the groin in a game of pickup basketball.

We need to reexamine why this is all so amusing. Is it because men are so unable to control their hormonal inclinations on Mexico City's Metro that they need to be penned off? Is it because men are intrinsically better at presiding over households that "leftover women" in China have every reason to be anxious? Is it because men are incorrigibly unreliable sex partners that birth control should be produced only for women? If men have an inborn urge to commit rape, is US vice president Mike Pence right not to eat alone with any woman who is not his wife? If so, maybe Mrs. Pence should be wary of dinner dates herself.

If testosterone really is the elixir of manly achievement, shouldn't we be dosing our boys from birth? If untethered misogyny is deep-rooted in men, is Donald Trump merely revealing the id underneath all the other, more genteel leaders? If sexual exploitation and abuse by UN peacekeepers shows men reverting to their involuntary sexual and aggressive drives, should women-only contingents form all UN missions?

The #MeToo movement gained widespread visibility in 2017 on a surge of rage, powered by women who had been sexually abused, assaulted, and harassed by men. If we choose to embrace the idea that attacking women is central to men's entrenched instincts and identity, the battle has no winners. If we accept that violence is a core feature rather than a flaw of male behavior, and that assault is men's essential nature reasserting itself, we cripple our ability to identify and combat misogyny, gender bias, and discrimination. The day we see a boy or a man kicked in the balls and it is not funny, we will know we've made some progress.

We can do better, and we need to ask more from modern masculinities. We owe it to our daughters, our sons, and ourselves to reeducate our brains, our institutions, and our public policy to recognize that men are so much more capable and complex than today's summary judgments on the biology of masculinity would have us believe.

ACKNOWLEDGMENTS

I T'S REALLY NOT THE SAME AT ALL, BUT WRITING BOOKS IS PROBABLY the closest I will ever come to being pregnant and giving birth. The gestation in this case takes years and is likewise always idiosyncratic, a marvelous brew of agitation, worry, and wonder. Like human conception, a book is a joyfully joint enterprise. My debt is great to many colleagues, friends, and family members who have accompanied me in the course of this project, which was originally conceived as a presentation at the Chicago Humanities Festival in 2013. The theme that year was "Animals." After initially responding, "I don't do animals," it occurred to me that, well, perhaps I do.

For their insights, cajoling, invitations to lecture, reading of drafts, every manner of critique, and friendship throughout the period this book came to life, my thanks to Mickey Ackerman, Elia Aguilar, Josefina Alcazar, Sara Amin, Peter Andreas, Non Arkaraprasertkul (王光亮), Miguel Armenta, Omar Awan, Roger Bartra, Victoria Bernal, Federico Besserer, Po Bhattacharyya, Stanley Brandes, Lundy Braun, Susan Brownell, Matti Bunzl, Cai Yifeng (蔡一峰), Sylvia Chant, Nitsan Chorev, Beshara Doumani, Fan Ke (范可), Paja Faudree, Anne Fausto-Sterling, Michael Flood, William Freedberg, Lina Fruzzetti, Agustín Fuentes, Frances Hasso, Patrick Heller, Gilbert Herdt, Lung-hua Hu (胡龍華), Marcia Inhorn, Dan Kahn, Sarah Kahn, Mark Kepple, David Kertzer,

Tim Kessler, Max Kohlenberg, Louise Lamphere, Bradley Levinson, Minhua Ling, Tanya Luhrmann, Catherine Lutz, Rolf Malungo de Souza, Alice Mandel, Clara Mantini-Briggs, Hannah Marshall, Katherine Mason, Michelle McKenzie, Bob Mercer, Shaylih Muehlmann, Nefissa Naguib, Lynne Nakano, Robin Nelson, Ruben Oliven, Sherry Ortner, Pan Tianshu (天舒), Ernesto Persechino, David Rand, Lucía Rayas, Clara Eugenia Rojas Blanco, Noha Sadek, Robert Sapolsky, Nancy Scheper-Hughes, Shao Jing (邵京), Susan Short, Daniel Smith, Michael Steinberg, Edward Steinfeld, Sun Huizhu (孙惠柱), Ivonne Szasz, Josh Taub, Brendan Thornton, Lingzhen Wang (王玲珍), Wang Mengqi, Angela Wai-ching Wong, Ken Wong, and Carol Worthman.

I became friends with several of the people named above when I contacted them because I didn't agree with arguments they had made and I wanted to discuss our diverging perspectives. In some cases, I still don't go along with their thinking; but in the book I do try to engage sincerely with them, and I am especially appreciative of their patience in trying to help me understand why I am the one who's still mistaken. Long may such dialogues thrive.

I offer special recognition of two individuals who for several decades have been essential in establishing and guiding the academic field of feminist men and masculinities studies. Michael Kimmel and Raewyn Connell have made inequality the center of these studies, as they inspired new generations of scholars and activists. Your global impact has been profound conceptually and institutionally and I have enormously benefited from your counsel and assistance.

For granting me interviews—the best were really conversations—in the course of this research, my appreciation especially to Sául Alveano, Daniel Armenta, Miguel Armenta, Richard Bribiescas, Martha Delgado, Frans de Waal, Fili Fernández, Tina Garnanez, Deborah Gordon, Sarah Blaffer Hrdy, Li Gangwu (李刚吾), Norma López, Daniel Morales, Demond Mullins, Richard Rosenthal, Marcos Ruvalcaba, Gabriel Saavedra, Henry Tricks, Yang Luxia (杨璐瑕), and Zhu Wenbing (朱文彬).

To Brown University undergraduates who assisted with transcription, bibliographic research, statistical analysis, and language tips, your help was invaluable: Kevin Dhali, Drew Hawkinson, Silvina Hernández, Iván Hofman, Paula Martínez Gutiérrez, Alan Mendoza Sosa, Max Song, Brenton Stokes, Daphne Xu, and Wen (Elaine) Wen (闻雯).

To my agent Gail Ross and all her team, especially Dara Kay and Katie Zanecchia, your enthusiasm and vision for the project were key. To TJ Kelleher, who first brought the book to Basic; Eric Hanney, who improved the argument in each chapter; Kaitlin Carruthers-Busser for handling production; Katherine Streckfus for superb copyediting; and everyone else at Basic, from editing to promotion, my deep thanks.

Thanks also to audiences for their questions and comments, especially in Chicago, Ciudad Juárez, Durham, Hong Kong, Irvine, London, Los Angeles, Mexico City, Nanjing, New Haven, New York City, Oslo, Porto Alegre, Providence, Rio de Janeiro, São Paulo, Shanghai, Suva, Vancouver, and Wollongong. I am grateful as well for the Brown China Initiative and for Brown University research funds that provided critical financial support.

My deepest appreciation to my children, Maya Gutmann-McKenzie and Liliana Gutmann-McKenzie: you define the best of life. To Nancy O'Connor and Bob O'Connor, for the best of times. To Ana Amuchástegui, Charles Briggs, and Ángeles Clemente, *por estar presentes, siempre*. To my mother, Ann Oliver, and my cousin Debby Rosenkrantz, for the moral compasses you show in life.

And to Deborah Kahn, for your infinite grace, compassion, and rock-steady character. I am beholden to you in all ways.

My brothers, Rick Goldman and Rob Goldman, have had my back since I was three, and that has never changed. Together with treasured friends Todd Winkler, Jeffrey Lesser, Pedro Lewin, Paco Ferrándiz, and Terry Hopkins, for decades you have each shown me how to live as a good man, a good father, a good husband, and a good person. I'm not big on the concept of male bonding, but you are my menschen, and I dedicate this book to you with my love and gratitude.

NOTES

INTRODUCTION

1. As will become obvious, often in these endnotes I delve into more scholarly tangents and recondite matters. In addition to providing references, my purpose is to expand discussion of less essential but still intriguing points; to give the original of a term that I have translated from another language; and to offer special thanks to specific colleagues who have suggested a particular interpretation, example, or quotation. I hope the notes will be helpful, suggestive, and entertaining.

For the *Newsweek* article, see Dovy 2018. The original scientific paper is "Negative Correlation Between Salivary Testosterone Concentration and Preference for Sophisticated Music in Males," by Doi et al. 2018. The purpose of the academic study was "to clarify the biological basis of individual differences in music preference." Hormones were the biological factor of choice. The researchers could not explain why they found no correlation between testosterone levels and music preference in thirty-nine women. Despite the fact that the original study lumped classical, world, and jazz music together under the category of "sophisticated," it's anybody's guess as to why *Newsweek* selected jazz and not classical as the "sophisticated music" linked to low levels of testosterone. Could it be that jazz in the United States is more associated with African Americans and classical with whites?

2. I sometimes use the term "we" loosely in this book, a shorthand way of discussing ideas and activities that are widespread although not universal. Academic texts usually shun such sweeping inclusiveness. But a central

point I am trying to make is that more of us share fallacious beliefs about men and masculinity than we might like to admit, so let's not disregard the possibility of our own involvement in problematic approaches to maleness.

3. Bruni 2016; Isaacson 2017; Parker 2010; Bernstein 2017; Blow 2017; Burke 2016, 28.

4. As far as I can tell, the term "biobabble" comes from Krugman 1997.

5. Sapolsky 2005, 49.

6. Vargas Llosa 1978, 8.

7. I should perhaps qualify this statement: the anthropologist of war Brian Ferguson (personal communication) believes there is evidence in the Black Sea, Dahomey, and other regions of ancient groups of women warriors. The fact remains that in none of these instances were women ruling society overall.

8. My thanks to Michael Kimmel for this insight.

9. "Search for the ideal man": *xunzhao nanzihan*, 寻找男子汉. The adage in Chinese is *Gou gaibuliao chi shi*, 狗改不了吃屎. My thanks again to Mengqi Wang for suggesting this expression to me.

I debated leaving out the Chinese characters and transliterations of Chinese terms and names in this book. After all, with a little work and ingenuity those who know Chinese could figure out the original Chinese on their own. And then I traveled back to China and was again struck by the amount of English that is found on street signs, shops, metros, elevator speakers, restaurants, and newspapers. All this has no doubt made English just a little less daunting for those in China who have never formally studied it. I decided that if readers found the Chinese characters too annoying, they could easily skip over them. We English speakers need to grow more accustomed to foreign tongues and writing. After all, who could read the following Chinese banners along the sidelines at the World Cup 2018? «万达» «激光电视中国领先»

So, in the spirit of "Okja" and submersing oneself in foreign languages, to the more adventurous reader, I ask you to spend a little time looking at the characters. They won't bite, and you might even make a bit of sense of them with practice. That said, they're mostly in the endnotes.

10. On Uganda, see Heald 1999; on Europe, see Laqueur 1990.

CHAPTER 1: GENDER CONFUSION

1. Kimmel 1994, 131 (emphasis in original).

2. Trump tweeted on July 26, 2018, 5:55 a.m. and 6:04 a.m.: "After consultation with my Generals and military experts, please be advised that the

United States Government will not accept or allow . . . [t]ransgender individuals to serve in any capacity in the U.S. Military."

3. Take these examples: "People in the United States no longer know how to change a sparkplug." You have to remind yourself that "people" means just men. Or, "Bengals fans decided that they should bring their children and leave the wives at home" (where "fans" really means "male fans"). Or, "A majority of professors voted to admit their female colleagues as members of the faculty club" (where "professors" really means "male professors"). On the terms "marked" and "unmarked," see Waugh 1982.

4. Rubin 1984, 4.

5. Best-selling author Jordan Peterson was an inspiration to incels during this period. See Peterson 2018.

6. See Marks 2015, 91.

7. Hofstadter 1992 [1944], 204. It is no coincidence that Hofstadter was involved in radical left political activities in his youth.

8. See Milam 2019, 7–8.

9. De Beauvoir 1970 [1949], 29. Not accidentally, de Beauvoir titled her first chapter "The Data of Biology."

10. Wilson 2000 [1975], 547. Notably, Anne Harrington writes that in the 1980s psychiatry in the United States became a biological discipline. See Harrington 2019. Wilson claims feminist credentials of sorts. As a reporter for the *Wall Street Journal* wrote in 2014, quoting Wilson, "'Ants don't offer any good moral lessons or any lessons about organization,' he says. 'All ants that you see are female, and you know, I'm an ardent feminist, but that's feminism run amok.' Male ants are allowed to be with females only for a short time. 'They have only one function in the colony and in life itself, which you don't want to expatiate in The Wall Street Journal,' he says with a smile." See Wolfe 2014.

11. Wilson 2004 [1978], x, 38.

12. Prum 2017, 81.

13. I regret that I am not exaggerating how far Wilson extended his purview. On the second page of his 697-page book, he explicitly criticizes the views about biology (and "socialism") raised by "Marxists," "Old Marxists," and the "New Left" (2000 [1975], vi). Contra a basic tenet of every brand of feminism, Wilson also argues that "even with identical education for men and women and equal access to all professions, men are likely to maintain disproportionate representation in political life, business, and science" (2004 [1978]:103). Many have made this point about the politics and science of these white southerners and northern Jews, including, recently, Sapolsky 2017, 384.

14. On the muxe', see, especially, Miano Borruso 2002 and Stephen 2002.

15. Cited in Miano Borruso 2002, 149.

16. Among his many publications on the Sambia, see Herdt 1994.

17. Herdt 1994, 3, 304.

18. On the hijras, see, especially, Reddy 2005.

19. Marx 1977 [1844].

20. Pinker 2002, 351.

21. See Pinker 2002. We will look more closely at this and other analyses of rape in Chapter 5.

22. King James Version.

23. It goes without saying that the Southern Baptists are hardly alone in insisting that men lead and women follow. Catholics do not have female priests any more than Orthodox Jews, with rare exceptions, have women rabbis.

24. See Fausto-Sterling et al. 2015. Though this is a study of mothers and infants, I am confident that its conclusions would apply perhaps even more to fathers and infants.

CHAPTER 2: THE SCIENCE OF MALENESS

1. The numbers are an approximation as there is little regulation in this industry. In 2014, *Time* magazine ran an article by David Von Drehle, "Manopause?! Aging, Insecurity and the $2 Billion Testosterone Industry." See Von Drehle 2014.

2. On the history of sex hormone research and its applications, I draw especially on Oudshoorn 1994 and 2003 and Fausto-Sterling 2000.

3. Especially helpful in understanding the science and social implications of testosterone are Hoberman 2005 and Sapolsky's essay "The Trouble with Testosterone" (in Sapolsky 1997) and his 2017 magnum opus *Behave: The Biology of Humans at Our Best and Worst*. See also the very different treatments in Fine 2017; Herbert 2015; and Morgentaler 2009.

4. As for warning labels, the marketing firm Global Industry Analysts advises, in its 203-page report of February 2018, that there are "growing concerns over cardiovascular risk of TRT," and that such heart problems could represent "a key challenge to growth" of TRT in all global markets. The firm is also surprisingly quiet in responding to popular beliefs about testosterone, especially that higher levels of the hormone may cause more aggressive behavior and sexual predation by men. Regardless, sales have boomed because of the growing sense among older men that their happi-

ness and value are tied to maintaining youthful bodies. See Global Industry Analysts, Inc., 2018.

5. Hoberman 2005, 25, 27.

6. Herbert 2015, 22.

7. Oudshoorn 1994, 17.

8. Sapolsky 1997.

9. In his benchmark 2006 survey of the scientific literature on testosterone, British endocrinologist John Archer writes, "There is a weak and inconsistent correlation between testosterone levels and aggression in [human] adults, and . . . administration of testosterone to volunteers typically does not increase their aggression." See Archer 2006, 320. Just to make matters more complicated, neuroscientist Lise Eliot writes that "growing evidence suggests that the neurotransmitter serotonin is actually a better marker than testosterone for aggression and violence" (2009, 269).

10. See discussion in Sapolsky 2017, 106. Biological anthropologists are largely in accord with these conclusions. Primatologist Agustín Fuentes, for instance, notes that "testosterone itself is not associated in any causal way with increased aggressive behavior or in the patterns of the exhibition of aggression" (2012, 143). Richard Bribiescas writes that "increases in testosterone are not associated with greater aggression or libido," adding that the range of testosterone levels among American men is "quite extreme, with tenfold differences between the highest and lowest men without any apparent pathological effects" (2006, 132, 169).

11. Eliot 2009, 268.

12. Herbert 2015, 116–118, 143, 194.

13. See Alex Jones's advertising on his InfoWars store website for men interested in "Super Male Vitality."

14. Hershatter 1996, 90.

15. Furthermore on the biology of Low T, it is important to remember that what "low" means is always relative to some other "high." In the United States, the lows of men in their fifties and beyond are being compared to the highs of men in their twenties. On average, the testosterone levels of men in the United States begin declining in their thirties by approximately 1 percent per year, or roughly 10 percent per decade. This process is directly correlated with greater rates of obesity as men age. This much is known. But also notable is the fact that although average testosterone levels drop for men in the United States, this is not universally true. In studies among pastoralists in Kenya, for instance, average levels remain far more constant for men into

old age. (My thanks to Benjamin Campbell for help in understanding how and why testosterone levels are different in older men in different countries and nutritional settings. For more information, see Campbell et al. 2006.)

What all this means—for sexual interest and abilities, energy levels, and more—is debatable. Men grow more obese, and for some reason they don't realize that their more sedentary lives and worsening diets could be leading factors in simultaneously decreasing their energy and libido. Yet, instead of altering their diet and activities to offset these changes in physiology, a growing number of men in the United States have resorted to seeking medical boosts to their testosterone levels: most of those who do (60 percent) use gels they wipe into their armpits, whereas 25 percent prefer injections and another 12 percent apply patches.

16. Richardson 2013, 201. My discussion of genetics, genomics, and sex differences is guided by this study.

17. See Jordan-Young 2010, 79; Richardson 2013, 225.

18. Oates 1988, 69–70.

19. Bartra 2014, 180.

20. Hofstadter 1992 [1944], 164.

21. Duden and Samerski 2007, 168.

22. Fausto-Sterling 1992, 269.

23. Raine 2013, 33; Connell 2000, 22.

24. Cooper and Smith 2011, 9; United Nations Office on Drugs and Crime 2014, 11.

25. Ibid., 85.

26. And, of course, like-minded scientists squabble even among themselves. Joe Herbert writes about digit ratios that "lesbian women overall have more male-like ratios than heterosexual ones. But in males there is no difference between gay and straight men" (2015, 51).

27. Raine 2013, 194–198. Importantly, the 2D:4D hypothesis may be headed for the archives. Recent meta-analysis surveying all major scientific work on this conjecture concluded, "We find no evidence of 2D:4D better predicting aggression at different levels of risk" (Hönekopp and Watson 2011, 381); see also Wong and Hines 2016. My thanks to Agustín Fuentes for guiding me to these two papers.

Another whole line of inquiry darts between humans and other primates to draw out evolutionary lessons on the origins of male violence. We will review the accuracy and utility of such comparisons more closely in Chapter 3.

28. Austen 2016.

29. See Marks 2002 on the significance or not of "shared DNA."

CHAPTER 3: MONKEY SEE, HUMAN DO

1. One could also draw parallels to Kwame Anthony Appiah's discussion of identity, comparing Enlightenment thinkers with those who lump together and see the common humanity in all of us, versus those who stress identity politics and in this way, according to Appiah, overstate differences between people. See Appiah 2018.

2. My thanks to Gail Mummert for reminding me that "ox" (*buey*) here has a double meaning: as a beast of burden and as a fool.

3. "Part Man, Part Monkey," by Bruce Springsteen. Copyright © 1998 Bruce Springsteen (Global Music Rights). Reprinted by permission. International copyright secured. All rights reserved.

4. See Pierson 2005.

5. Leach 1964, 152. Regarding Leach, then again, perhaps the matter is more one of longing. As John Berger famously wrote in *Why Look at Animals?*, "In the last two centuries, animals have gradually disappeared. Today we live without them. And in this new solitude, anthropomorphism makes us doubly uneasy" (2009, 21).

In Spanish, goats are *cabrones*; dogs are *perros*; donkeys are *burros*; pigs are *cochinos*; rats are *ratas*; a beast is a *bestia*; a cow a *vaca*; a slut a *zorra*; and worms are *gusanos*.

The Chinese: duck, *ya*, 鸭; chicken, *ji*, 鸡. For those interested, there are various theories as to why men here might be compared to ducks and women to chickens. The most likely, if least salacious, is that a homophone for chicken (*ji*) is used in more formal expressions for female prostitutes (娼 妓 and 妓 女, *changji* and *jinü*); if so, "duck" could simply be part of the wordplay with another familiar fowl. Also in Chinese, dinosaurs, *konglong*, 恐龙; frogs, *wa*, 蛙; a turtle egg, *wangbadan*, 王八蛋; and monkeys, *houzi*, 猴子.

6. See, especially, Darwin 2009 [1872]. Descartes's term was *bête-machine*.

7. Milam 2019, 227.

8. Translational sticklers object to this rendering of Lévi-Strauss, insisting that the closer translation would be "Animals are good to think." The original French reads, "Les espèces sont choisies non comme bonnes à manger, mais comme bonnes à penser." In English, see Lévi-Strauss 1971 [1963], 89. And if you want to get even sticklier, really, "espèces" literally means "species" in English, though this is often translated (in context) to mean "animals."

Our deeply obsessive, sometimes neurotic, and perhaps even incestuous relationship with nonhuman animals had also already caught the attention of Sigmund Freud, who wrote about totemism and human-animal affiliations in a long-discredited lumping of "savages and neurotics." See Freud 1990 [1913].

9. Nagel 1974. Then there's the fanciful comparison made by Jordan Peterson (2018, 7) between humans and lobsters. The commonalities? Men and lobsters need territory and safe hiding places, are sometimes soft and vulnerable, and, "like Clint Eastwood in a spaghetti Western," sometimes wave their arms about to look tall and dangerous. If you try hard enough, you can compare men to anything.

10. Albee 2000, especially 80, 82, and 86 (emphasis in original). Edward Albee's Martin was drawn into his human-animal-divinity love affair through the eyes of Sylvia the goat. Getting naked with Sylvia was how Martin expressed his devotion to the goat. Perhaps Albee's tableau is not markedly dissimilar from a notorious scene described by philosopher Jacques Derrida (2002, 372), when the Frenchman was confronted naked by a pet cat. The sage reported his deep shame before "the insistent gaze of the animal."

11. De Waal 2001, 295.

12. De Waal 2013, 12.

13. See also Richard Prum's delightful discussion of the variability of ape sex in his *Evolution of Beauty* (2017).

14. Interview with Frans de Waal by author, March 10, 2014, Yerkes Laboratory, Atlanta, Georgia.

15. Interview, March 10, 2014.

16. De Waal 1999, 260.

17. Interview, March 10, 2014.

18. Hrdy 2000, 80.

19. Hrdy 2009, 3; interview with Sarah Hrdy by author, May 5, 2014, La Citrona Farms, Winters, California. She also writes, "The last outstanding distinction between us and other apes involves a curious packet of hyper-social attributes that allow us to monitor the mental states and feelings of others" (2009, 9).

20. Hrdy 2009, 162, 168.

21. Jordan-Young 2010, 118.

22. See Zuk 2002, 51.

23. See Hrdy 2000, 82, referring to Hrdy 1981.

24. Hrdy 2000, 92, 90.

25. Prum 2017, 277 (emphasis in original).

26. Fuentes 2012, 14.

27. King James Version.

28. One of the more cited sources is Larry L. Wolf's 1975 "'Prostitution' Behavior in a Tropical Hummingbird," in which he writes, "Since sexual behavior in these cases is being used for [sic] an energetic benefit for the female, I term this 'prostitution' behavior." Would it be unfair to ask what Wolf knows about human prostitution? At least he had the good graces to put "prostitution" in scare quotes. On harems, this word is used by virtually every primatologist, although they appear to know nothing of human harems and have encountered only primates whose dominant males have sex with many females. The notion that this arrangement was completely one-sided, "in favor" of the males, and that these same females were having sex only with the alpha male, turns out in many instances to have been an artifact of primatologist bias and not what was occurring on the ground. Nonetheless, now that we have untold documentation of female primates having sex with many males (and not a few females), no one, as far as I know, talks of females manipulating harems of males. That would apparently just spoil the salacious (covetous?) fun of our human male observers. A standard text used to compare male mallard ducks and humans is Barash 1980.

29. Prum 2017, 172–173 (emphasis in original).

30. Pinker 2002, 163.

31. See Marks 2002, 29.

32. De Waal 1999, 258.

33. De Waal 2013, 60 (emphasis in original). For a discussion of this issue for general readers, see de Waal 2016, 26; for a more academic analysis, see de Waal 1999.

34. For a searing exposé on exaggerated analogies between ant and human behavior, see Gordon 2010, 1, 4. Gordon is a biologist of ants.

35. De Waal 2016, 13.

36. Gould 1995, 433.

37. In response to reading a journal article sharply critiquing anthropomorphism in microbiology (Davies 2010), a student of mine wrote that microbes "most likely" don't have a sense of agency, revealing again the allure of biological explanations (and my failure as a teacher).

CHAPTER 4: THE MALE LIBIDO

1. Eliot 2009, 300.

2. I went to talk with my colleague about the slides and learned that he had removed the one with cheerleaders from the latest version of the lecture, and that the whole football players / cheerleaders finale had been

used mainly to prompt discussion and debate among the students. I raised my concerns about overdrawn parallels and we agreed to continue discussing these issues.

3. Spain: Brandes 1980; Morocco: Mernissi 1987; Indonesia: Heider 1976.

4. Among the many studies at the time that found differences between women and men in visual sexual stimuli, see Fisher and Byrne 1978 and Malamuth 1996. See also the history of the science of gendered visual stimulation in Jordan-Young 2010, Chapter 6.

5. See Eliot 2009 and Jordan-Young 2010 on all questions related to sex and the brain.

6. Bribiescas 2006, 83.

7. Eliot 2009, 15 (emphasis in original).

8. Fausto-Sterling 2000, 52 (and throughout). Estimates vary, but Fausto-Sterling says 1.7 percent of all births are intersex babies, adding that this can't be taken as an exact count (51). Ahmed and Rodie write, "Genital anomalies may occur as commonly as 1 in 300 births" (2010, 198). Either way, it is not an enormous percentage, and it could be argued therefore that intersexuality doesn't significantly impact the idea that there are two kinds of sex organs. But that would also be like saying because the number of redheads in the world is less than 2 percent, we should ignore them as in any way reflective of hair color. Which would be a shame.

9. Joel 2011, 2. See also Joel 2016.

10. See Laqueur 1990, esp. 150.

11. Eliot 2009, 5, 6 (emphasis in original).

12. See Hyde 2005, 590.

13. Arizpe 1990, xv.

14. McNamara 1974, 108. I have conducted research with Mexfam, the International Planned Parenthood Federation (IPPF) affiliate in Mexico, for decades, and I represent the third in four generations of my family to work with them. More details on the history of family planning, contraception, and indigenous midwives in Mexico are in Gutmann 2007.

15. The most famous is Octavio Paz's *Labyrinth of Solitude*, first published in 1949 and read by every generation of schoolchildren thereafter. It may be difficult for people from English-speaking countries to appreciate how one book could have been read by every literate person in a particular country. The only equivalent book that nearly everyone in the United States has read—and its content is not at all equivalent—might be *The Cat in the Hat*.

16. See Hirsch 2003. Hirsch and Nathanson (2001, 413) point out that withdrawal as a form of birth control has been incorrectly classified as a

"traditional" method (in contrast to "modern" methods). As they report, dichotomous taxonomies of traditional and modern don't do justice to the evocative contours that men and women who have practiced withdrawal use to describe it.

17. A program officer from the National Science Foundation, with whom I had some correspondence in the early 2000s on vasectomies in Mexico, informed me that he thought a research project on the subject was unnecessary, because one could easily correlate vasectomy rates to macho and non-macho cultures around the world. This was a culturalist a priori explanation that, if followed to its logical conclusion, would provide metrics for how macho a culture might be. In the United Kingdom at that time, 18 percent of men had supposedly been sterilized; in Mexico, the figure was closer to 2 percent. Therefore, I queried, did he think the UK was nine times less macho? At least his argument rested on grounds other than men's inherent biology.

18. Statistics are reprinted in Pile and Barone 2009, 298.

19. One sociodemographic factor did correlate to men's decision to get sterilized: *"paridad satisfecha,"* i.e., when a man decided he had as many children as he wanted.

20. See Viveros 2002 on the study of vasectomies and men's sexual and reproductive health generally in Latin America.

21. Sprinkle children around: *dejar hijos regados.*

22. On the sterilization campaign in India, see, especially, Gwatkin 1979 and Tarlo 2003, as well as Mistry's brilliant 1997 novel *A Fine Balance.*

23. My friend told me she had not heard about Freud's famous essay on the "Wolf Man" that recounted a similar historical basis for infantile neurosis. See Freud 1995 [1918].

24. Jordan-Young 2010, 132.

CHAPTER 5: MEN'S NATURAL AGGRESSIONS

1. In his 411 BC play, Aristophanes famously had women withhold sex until their men had found a way to make peace in the Peloponnesian War. Spike Lee (2015) did something similar to stop gang wars in Chicago in the time of the Iraq War. In response to the fascist advance in Spain in the 1930s, Virginia Woolf issued a feminist call to antiwar arms in *Three Guineas* (1938), asking how women could oppose the wars of men. In her essay on war photography, Susan Sontag (2002) concludes, "We can't imagine how dreadful, how terrifying war is—and how normal it becomes. Can't understand, can't imagine."

2. On gendered crime, violence, and aggression, see Kruttschnitt 2013 and Collins 2008; and on these issues and cross-cultural variation in male violence against women, see also Fuentes 2012 and Smuts 1992.

3. Smuts 1992, 31–32.

4. For a claim to the now largely discredited "selfish gene," see Dawkins 1976. Wrangham and Peterson (1996) write about demonic males, blurring boundaries in the name of cross-species male esprit de corps. The role of the rise of agriculture in the decline of humanity is discussed in Diamond 1999. Carl von Clausewitz (1989 [1832]) argued that war should be understood less as unique and more as the militarized projection of politics.

5. This is a rough count, because a number of countries have qualified conscription, such as in case of emergencies or when the ranks cannot be filled by volunteers. Conscription is not enforced in some of these countries, and often there are mechanisms, such as lotteries, that select only a percentage of eligible young men. In many countries, there are legal exemptions and ways for wealthier youths to avoid participation in military life.

6. Among those required to register are "undocumented [male] immigrants" and "U.S. citizens or immigrants who are born male and have changed their gender to female." On the other hand, "individuals who are born female and have changed their gender to male" are exempt from registering for a possible future draft by the US military. In other words, if you are male and between eighteen and twenty-five years old, and you sneak across the US-Mexican border, risking life and limb, *coyote* smugglers, and *La Migra*, upon arriving on the northern side of the international divide you are expected to dash off as quickly as you can to register for the draft of the country that has done its best to prevent you from entering. Young men residing without papers in the United States are simultaneously subject to both deportation and conscription by the US government. And if you are a transwoman, the fact that a lot of people might have thought you were male at some earlier point trumps anything you might know about yourself, while your trans brothers can never be draft-ready because they do not meet some fixed notion of manhood, whether genital, chromosomal, or morphological.

7. Fuller versions of the stories of Tina and Demond can be found in Gutmann and Lutz 2010, which is based on the oral histories of six antiwar veterans.

8. Years later he was able to return to school and finish a PhD in sociology at the City University of New York. In 2013, Demond began as an assistant professor at Indiana University of Pennsylvania.

9. Herbert 2015, 147, 148.

10. Bribiescas 2006, 143, 222, 223. See also Bribiescas et al. 2012.

11. Brown 2014, 132.

12. Awori et al. 2013, 3.

13. Zeid 2005. I was part of a team that conducted interviews on SEA in 2007 with UN peacekeepers in Haiti, Lebanon, and Kosovo.

14. Interview with Daniel Morales, Port-au-Prince, Haiti, February 27, 2007.

15. Pinker 2002, 162 (emphasis in original).

16. And rarely does an intellectual and his scholarship get the praise and endorsement from influential corporate movers and shakers that Pinker has received from Bill Gates. See, for example, Galanes 2018.

17. Martin 2003, 378, critiquing Thornhill and Palmer 2000.

18. Joanna Bourke points out with respect to rape, "It is not simply that the statistics are not collected in a consistent or reliable manner. They cannot exist" (2007, 15).

19. Sanday 2003, 357. See also Kimmel 2003.

20. Herbert 2015, 101; Bourke 2007, 178.

21. Pinker 2002, 164, 162, 359–360, 369, 362.

22. Kipnis 2017, 8 (emphasis in original). Furthermore, Kipnis (2017, 14) called attention to one underexamined assumption in discussions of rape culture, namely, an underlying ethos that "men need to be policed, women need to be protected. If rape is the norm, then male sexuality is by definition predatory; women are, by definition, prey," and women's agency is effectively undermined.

23. Thornhill and Palmer 2000, 67. Why most poor men do not rape, well that is supposedly a mystery. Why rape rates vary from society to society and region to region is likewise evidently mysterious. One way to get around the thorny problem of not being able to back up any of these claims with hard evidence is, as many have noted, the invocation of the almighty conditional. To take a random page from the Thornhill and Palmer book, we read, "One *probable* reason why such men are *likely* . . . ," "physical attractiveness in men *may* have connoted . . . ," women "*may* receive few material benefits . . . ," "The female's strategy *might* . . . ," "This display *may* . . . ," "which *may* increase the man's perception . . . ," "*may* result in . . . ," "*If* a woman's display . . . ," "*would* involve testing . . . ," "*could* be explored empirically." All of which "calls for further research" (2000, 70, emphasis added). To which we can only add, Amen to that.

24. If only what Patty Gowaty declared in 2010 were true: "Because of the important differences between rape and forced copulations, those of us

who study animal behavior agreed years ago to refer to 'forced copulation' in non-human animals, and to reserve the term 'rape' for humans" (2010, 760).

25. In order, Bekiempis 2015; Kingkade 2015; Filipovic 2015; "Many US College Men Deny" 2015; Culp-Ressler 2015 (emphasis in original). The academic in me can't resist a few corrections: nowhere do the authors of the original study state where the students they studied were enrolled; the authors of the report did not all teach at the University of North Dakota; and for a subsequent news article in 2017, albeit on International Women's Day that year, to talk about a 2014 study as "new" is a bit of a stretch. The scholarly article the news items refer to is Edwards et al. 2014.

26. Statistics here are culled from the National Sexual Violence Resource Center. See www.nsvrc.org/statistics, which is updated regularly.

27. See Sanday 1981, 2003.

28. It will be recalled that forty-nine of fifty states voted for Nixon in 1972. Only Massachusetts and the District of Columbia voted for the Democratic candidate, George McGovern.

29. Bender 1970.

30. Some estimates state that as many as 90 percent of women in the United States will at some time suffer from premenstrual syndrome (PMS), and a much smaller number, perhaps 2–5 percent of these women, will regularly be wracked with the most severe symptoms, known as premenstrual dysphoric disorder (PMDD). Legal claims in the United States, the United Kingdom, France, Australia, and other countries have been made in recent years arguing that women who experienced PMS or PMDD during an illegal act should be exonerated or given lighter punishments because of their disorder. Although generally unsuccessful in getting clients entirely off for various crimes, including those involving violent outbursts directly linked by the lawyers to PMS and PMDD, these pleas may have resulted in lighter sentences.

Lawyers in these cases often declared that their clients' PMS caused changed mental states, and because they did not have the requisite *mens rea*, or guilty intent, they should not be charged for the crimes committed. With PMDD becoming a full-fledged syndrome in *DSM-V* beginning in 2013, lawyers arguing for insanity, diminished capacity, or especially mitigating factors could offer greater legal foundation and could enjoy greater success.

There are serious questions to be raised as to whether the newly sanctified category of PMDD represents a step forward or a circling back to earlier concerns with women and hysteria. It's hard not to be concerned that women are being stuffed back into the emotions-out-of-control box. "Each time the defense is accepted," writes physician Laura Downs in recounting feminist fears about PMS claims in legal cases, "it lends credence to the characterization of women as creatures driven by hormonal whims" (2002, 6).

It is difficult to point to a correlation between menstrual cycles and aberrant behavior without sliding down the slippery slope to generalizing about women being unable to control their biological processes, their "hormonal limitations," whether gynecological, endocrinological, or mental. In the workplace, in divorce hearings, and in the political arena, stigma and stereotyping associating women's physiology with the uncontrollable leads to discrimination against, exclusion of, and inequality for women.

My thanks to my student Silvina Hernández for her research on PMS. Studies on legal cases involving PMS defenses include Press 1983; Lewis 1990; Solomon 1995; and Downs 2002.

31. United Nations Office on Drugs and Crime 2014, 77.

32. See Lutz 2009.

33. "Transcript" 2016.

34. The line by Xi (2012) in its original Chinese was: «Dang jing wu yiren shi nan'er, meishenma ren chulai kangzheng,» 但竟无一人是男儿，没什么人出来抗争. Xi's call to manliness had historical echoes as well for all assembled. During the tenth century in China there lived a concubine named Madame Huarui, also known as Consort Xu. She was a well-known poet when the dynasty of her emperor, Meng, was overthrown, and when she was asked by the new emperor, Taizu, to write a special verse to mark the dynastic succession, she is reported to have responded on the spot with a song:

> The king on the rampart flies the white flag
> (*junwang cheng shang shu jiangqi*, 君王城上豎降旗).
> Deep within the palace how could I know?
> (*qie zai shen gong na de zhi*, 妾在深宮那得知)
> One hundred forty thousand all disarmed!
> (*shisi wan renqi jie jia*, 十四萬人齊解甲)
> Among these was there not a single man?
> (*geng wu yige shi nan'er*, 更無一個是男兒)

My thanks to anthropologist Mengqi Wang for sharing this literary reference. The translation of the poem is by Anthony C. Yu (see Wikipedia entry for "Madame Huarui").

Elanah Uretsky has a delicious illustration of the trials manly men face in China: they must be able to handle the "heat" of life. On the menu at a restaurant in Kunming, China, she spots Manly Fried Rice (*nanzihan chaofan* [男子汉炒饭]). When Uretsky asks the proprietor of the establishment about the name, "she explained all the pressures contemporary Chinese men endure in their daily lives: 'They have family pressures (*jiating yali* [家庭压力]) and social pressures (*shehui yali* [社会压力]) that they deal with on a daily basis, which makes their lives very stressful. . . . A real *nanzihan* is a man who can eat such hot and spicy food without saying it's hot.'" Uretsky 2016, 54.

The term from Major General Luo Yuan (Luo 2010) was «Yanggang zhi qi, hulang zhi shi,» 阳刚之气，虎狼之师.

CHAPTER 6: I AM, THEREFORE I THINK

1. Tiger 1984 [1969], 208; see also Dyble et al. 2015.

2. See "Report of the Committee" 2017. See also William Domhoff's classic on the *Bohemian Grove and Other Retreats: A Study in Ruling-Class Cohesiveness*, 1975.

3. This leaves aside situations in which there are too few facilities for women.

4. See Kogan 2010, and more generally, on the topic of gender and bathrooms, the entire collection in which this work appears, edited by Molotch and Norén (2010).

5. Grossman 2009, 175.

6. If this happened with an ultra-orthodox Muslim man on a plane, would it make a difference in the public imagination? Islamophobia in the name of defending Muslim women against the tyranny of their men is a widespread hypocritical dogma in the United States and other countries.

7. That is, between *acoso* and *tocar*.

8. "Pushes against you with his shrimp": "Te arrima el camarón."

9. Curious counterexample to the brute behavior of riders on the subway at rush hour: when the large jitneys called *peseros* pack as many as fifty people on during rush hour, it's often easiest to board in the back, far away from the driver or assistant taking the fare. This then requires you to pass money forward, from hand to hand, involving as many as six or seven people, and if change is required, for it to come back the same way. One after another says, "Me lo pases" until the money reaches the driver. The politeness and consideration of strangers never fails, nor does the money ever fail to reach its recipient.

10. There are many scholarly writings in Mexico on men and masculinities. Among the ethnographies, reportage, and accounts that document the

lives of men in Mexico are Fernando Huerta's study of Volkswagen workers in Puebla (1999); Guillermo Núñez Noriega's work on male identities and intimacy in northern Mexico (2014); Rodrigo Parrini's study of male prisoners (2007); Carlos Monsiváis's chronicles of sexuality and affect in Mexico (1988); and my own books on a Mexico City squatter settlement (2006 [1996]) and men's sexual and reproductive health in Oaxaca (2007).

11. See Gutmann 2002, 229.

12. "Es molesto viajar aquí, pero no se compara con la violencia sexual que sufren las mujeres en sus traslados cotidianos." A video was available via CNN. See "'No es de hombres,' la compaña contra la violencia sexual que intrigó a México," CNN Español, March 31, 2017, cnnespanol.cnn .com/2017/03/31/no-es-de-hombres-la-campana-contra-la-violencia-sexual -que-intrigo-a-mexico.

13. "NoEsDeHombres Experimento Pantallas," YouTube, Primera Vuelta Tamaulipas, posted March 30, 2017, www.youtube.com/watch?v =5tngqqSUKBY.

14. See Brown 2006.

CHAPTER 7: FATHERING

1. Rich 1996, xi–xii.

2. Lewis 1963, 338; Yang 1945, 127–128. James Taggart reports the same kind of sleeping arrangements in the past in a rural area east of Mexico City, with "the youngest child sleeping with the mother on one mat, the father with one or two of the next youngest children on a second mat, and the other preadolescent children on as many other mats as are needed" (Taggart 1992, 78).

3. On this photo and several other anecdotes from Mexico City, see fuller discussions in Gutmann 2006 [1996].

4. See Hochschild 1989.

5. Mead 2001 [1928].

6. Parsons and Bales 1955.

7. On mother migrants and father left-behind caregivers in Southeast Asia, see Lam and Yeoh 2015; Thao 2015.

8. Quoted in Thao 2015, 146.

9. Luhrmann 2000, 8.

10. Prum 2017, 97. And, yes, I realize this is abusive anthropomorphism. I am not humorless when it comes to animal comparisons!

11. Birenbaum-Carmeli et al. 2015, 167, 168.

12. My thanks to my colleagues on the project, especially Lorena Santos, Anabel López, Ana Amuchástegui, Elyse Singer, and Florencia Barindelli, and to funding from the Virginia B. Toulmin Foundation.

13. Winnicott 1953.

CHAPTER 8: REVERTING TO NATURAL GENDERS IN CHINA

1. "Women Hold Up Half the Sky": «Funü neng ding banbiantian,» 妇女能顶半边天.

2. Zhang and Sun, 2014, 121.

3. Yang 1999, 50 65.

4. See Hong Fincher 2014; Davis 2010; Wang 2018.

5. Wang 2018, 87–88.

6. None of this is unique to China. Furious debates in the United States coinciding with the publication of *Lean In* by Sheryl Sandberg were echoed in China. Part of Sandberg's bestseller's appeal resided in the fact that she was the chief operating officer of Facebook. That affiliation was also coupled with anxieties experienced by younger women (and their parents) who wondered if women could "have it all," and what that might mean in real life. Sandberg's book was quickly translated into Chinese as *Xiangqian yibu*, 向前一步 (One step forward).

7. See Kam Louie's literary work on Chinese masculinities, in particular his emphasis on achievement in scholarship and the fine arts alongside the martial arts as the quintessence of manliness in particular historical periods in China. Louie 2002, 2016.

Especially helpful in thinking about the gender binary in modern China are Brownell and Wasserstrom 2002; Barlow 2004; and Davis and Friedman 2014. The quip about a "cult of chastity" is from Laqueur 2002, xiii.

8. A literate person in China is defined as someone knowing 2,000 characters in urban areas, and 1,500 characters in rural areas. Comparable figures for India, for example, were 18 percent in 1950 (close to China's rate) and 44 percent in 1981. Perhaps most telling, in India in 2011, literacy rates were 82 percent for men and 65 percent for women; in China by 2010, they had reached 98 percent for men and 93 percent for women.

By the 2010s, women slightly edged out men in student enrollment in higher education in China, although this was not true in the top-ranked universities.

9. This kind of "entertaining" is called *yingchou*, 应酬.

10. Zheng 2012, 653, 658. Zheng has written some of the best ethnographic studies on masculinity and contemporary prostitution in China. See also Zheng 2009a and 2009b; Johnson 2014.

11. Second Wife: *ernai,* 二奶; Little Third: *xiaosan,* 小三.

12. Three-High Women: *Sangaonü,* 三高女; "If You Are the One": *feicheng wurao,* 非诚勿扰; "I would rather cry in a BMW, than smile on a bike": «Wo ningyuan zuozai baomacheli ku, ye buyuanyi zuozai zixingcheshang xiao,» 我宁愿坐在宝马车里哭，也不愿意坐在自行车上笑.

13. *Hukou:* 户口.

14. Although it is often referred to in the Western press as the Shanghai Marriage Market, Blind Date Corner is a closer translation of the Chinese (*xiangqinjiao,* 相亲角) and carries fewer connotations of a sales transaction occurring. My preference for translating the spot as Blind Date Corner was solidified one Saturday in 2017, when I returned to Shanghai for a few days. As I strolled along the walkways of the park, a friendly young French man approached me and asked, in an almost conspiratorial, fellow-foreigner whisper, if I realized that women were being sold there. I thought he was making an ugly joke, but it seemed he was serious: he was taking the French, *marché du mariage,* quite literally.

My research at Blind Date Corner was made much easier through a collaboration with architect-anthropologist Non Arkaraprasertkul. We often wandered among the gawkers at Blind Date Corner, tag-team style. I warmed up the crowds with my hackneyed (and only semi-coherent) Chinese, and then Non stepped in to rescue the conversation and the ethnographic experience. Our animated conversations often gathered a pack of onlookers.

15. Regardless what you might have heard about yin-yang thinking, these terms are not reducible to neat female-male categories in Chinese philosophical traditions.

16. By 2018, Blind Date Corner was still thriving for parents, but for matchmakers it had become a more difficult venue. The municipal government had decided that making money on finding mates for parents would no longer be tolerated. As a result, matchmakers retreated into less conspicuous locations in the park, though they remained fairly easily identifiable by their thick notebooks in hand—parents sat empty-handed, as before, waiting and waiting for another parent to approach.

17. Wang 2016. "If You Are the One": *feicheng wurao,* 非诚勿扰; "One Out of a Hundred": *baili tiaoyi,* 百里挑一; "Luo Ji's Thinking": *Luo Ji siwei,* 罗辑思维; "Fatso Luo": *Luo Pangzi,* 罗胖子.

18. My wedding band never stopped tenacious matchmakers from asking, "Wouldn't you like a Chinese wife, too?"

19. "Just a pretty boy": *shuaiqi* vs. *shuai*, 帅气 vs. 帅; beauty: *piaoliang*, 漂亮; delicate in her manner: *qingxiu*, 清秀; proper in her conduct: *duanzheng*, 端正.

One popular advice columnist in China who goes by the nickname Ayawawa tries to help people understand the differences between men and women by a scale she has invented for "Mate Value": for men, this MV is established by his age, height, looks, wealth, IQ, EQ (emotional quotient), sexual capacity, and willingness to make a long-term commitment. For a woman, in ranking order, by her age, looks, height, bra cup size, weight, academic degrees, personality, and family background. See Kan 2017.

20. *Shizai qian tuo*, 实在欠妥. Xi's message was that "the majority of women will conscientiously shoulder the tasks of respecting the elders and loving the young, responsibility for educating their children, and assume their role in fostering family values" («Guangda funü yao zijue jianfu qi zun lao ai you, jiaoyu zinü de zeren, zai jiating meide jianshe zhong fahui zuoyong,» 广大妇女要自觉肩负起尊老爱幼、教育子女的责任，在家庭美德建设中发挥作用). Even using the rather antiquated term *funü* (妇女) was meant to elicit images of women from bygone eras. Sun Yatsen University feminist scholar Ai Xiaoming gathered responses to Xi's talk; see plus.google .com/109044788314125982317/posts/R3Hyy5uUn5T. My thanks to anthropologist Minhua Ling for bringing this speech and the reactions to my attention.

Also of note is the eager fascination people in Mexico, China, and other countries have in the Bill Clinton–Monica Lewinsky affair. One man in China told me he didn't understand the fuss in the United States over Bill and Monica: if (male) national leaders in China don't have "Second Wives," he assumed there was something wrong with them. In Mexico City back in the day, I remember having trouble getting friends to talk about anything else. Did I have any new dirt? Why was Bill stupid enough to get caught? Why did anyone other than Hillary care?

21. My thanks to my student Kevin Dhali for compiling the numbers on the flyers.

22. Leftover woman: *shengnü*, 剩女.

23. "Welcome to the Age of the Leftover Woman": «Huanying laidao shengnü shidai,» 欢迎来到剩女时代. *Cosmo* may have been inspired by a still earlier incarnation of the same derogatory idea here, the 2003 Japanese novel by Junko Sakai, *Makeinu no toboe* (The distant barking of losing dogs),

though in that case single women over thirty, "the losing dogs" of the title, were the objects of reflection. My thanks to anthropologist Minhua Ling for this reference.

24. "Outside the law": *feifa tongzhu*, 非法同住; "trial marriages": *shihun*, 试婚. Even the infamous gender ratio in China was evening out over time. In 2004, there were 121 boys for 100 girls; in 2015, 114 boys to 100 girls. Worldwide, the figure that year was 104 boys to 100 girls, so China still produced a flagrant disparity, but the trend was clearly moving in the direction of demography's so-called natural sex ratios.

25. Here and throughout this chapter I supplement my own fieldwork with the work of a range of scholars, including Hong Fincher 2014; Zhang and Sun 2014; and Merriman 2015.

26. "Leftover/Saintly Fighters": *sheng/sheng doushi*, 剩／圣斗士; "Leftovers Who Must Win": *bisheng/shengke*, 必剩／胜客; "Buddha's Leftovers from Fighting the Wars": *douzhan shengfo*, 斗战剩佛; "Great Leftover/Saint, Equal of Heaven": *qitian dasheng/sheng*, 齐天大剩／圣.

27. "Picky": *tiaoti*, 挑剔.

28. "Very high demands": *yaoqiu hen gao*, 要求很高.

29. "Their standards are too high": *biaozhun tai gao*, 标准太高; "serious inquiries only": *feicheng wurao*, 非诚勿扰 (the same as the TV show that is nonetheless usually translated into English as "If You Are the One").

CHAPTER 9: CAN WE CHANGE OUR BIOLOGY?

1. Quote from "Anthem" by Leonard Cohen, collected in *Stranger Music: Selected Poems and Songs*. Copyright © 1993 Leonard Cohen and Leonard Cohen Stranger Music, Inc., used by permission of The Wylie Agency LLC.

2. Curiously enough, in Mexico City AA is mainly for men; women suffering from the same afflictions are more likely to attend Narcotics Anonymous meetings, even if they are alcoholics and have never come near an opiate (see Brandes 2002). For more a more technical paper on alcoholism and ethnicity, and the following story of Jimmy and Dennis, see Gutmann 1999.

3. Martin 1994, 263.

4. Kolata 2012.

5. Fink 2017.

6. The symbolic relationship of guns and the phallus will not be rehearsed here, but it is not insignificant that one suggestive slang term for ejaculation in China literally means "to shoot like a canon" (*dapao*, 打炮).

7. Even when the killers don't fit the exact profile of young, male, and white, they usually fit two of the three categories and their killings fit social profiles. The person who slaughtered fifty-eight people in Las Vegas in 2017 was sixty-four years old but was white and male. The person who murdered forty-nine people in Orlando in 2016 identified himself as Afghan but was young and male.

8. For a recent academic discussion of fetishes (that unsurprisingly bears a strong resemblance to Karl Marx's thoughts on "commodity fetishism"), see Graeber 2005.

9. Keller 2010.

10. See Lancaster 2003 for a dissection of the search for the gay gene. For an influential scientific study on the "discovery" of the gay gene, see Hamer and Copeland 1994. Important ethnographies of men who have sex with men include Núñez-Noriega 2014 and Parker 1998.

11. Several of these broader points apply also in India, where Western biomedicine and Indian Ayurvedic medicine are practiced in often very integrated ways today.

12. On questions of TCM discussed in this section, see, especially, Farquhar 2002 and Zhang 2015. Quotes from Farquhar 2002, 64, 67, 235.

13. Quotes on impotence, TCM, and biomedicine in China are in Zhang 2015, 185, 173, 186.

14. When it comes to beliefs about the spirits of ancestors coming back to disturb descendants, the experience of my friends in Mexico City is not unique. One famous example studied by anthropologists is found among the Acholi of Northern Uganda, where unhappy spirits of the dead, known as *cen*, are said to "haunt the clan and its new children for generations." The beliefs have been especially prominent during civil war, the AIDS epidemic, and mass displacements (Finnström 2008, 192).

15. Marks 2015, 87. Marks was making a broader point about bodies in general rather than in their gendered qualities, but it applies just as well here.

16. Lock 2012, 129. For academic papers on the social implications of epigenetics, see also Lock 2013, 2015, and 2018 as well as Richardson 2017. See Lock and Palsson 2016 for an accessible presentation on the social implications of the new field of epigenetics. Prior to 1995, they note, the annual number of publications with "epigenetics" in their titles stood at less than 100. By 2010, there were 20,000. While the growth in the number of articles about testosterone reflects mainly changing social and political currents reducing men to their hormones (see Chapter 2 of this book), the growth in the number of articles about epigenetics represents the emergence of a new

field of inquiry that is taking biology by storm. The key, harkening back to Lamarck, is its renewed appreciation for the lasting impact of environmental factors interacting with human bodies.

17. See Lock and Palsson 2016 for a more thorough examination of these issues. For an influential paper on these themes, see Scheper-Hughes and Lock 1987.

18. Lock and Palsson 2016, 8–9, 79 (emphasis in original).

19. Richardson 2017, 32. Richardson also cautions that while epigenetics holds this promise, it has yet to be realized by those conducting basic epigenetics research.

CHAPTER 10: DON'T LET MEN OFF THE HOOK

1. See Peterson 2018, 51.

2. "Paradoxically, while sex is a biological category in a way that race is not, sex and gender are understood to be more open to choice and change than are race and ethnicity" (Brubaker 2016, 6).

3. My thanks to two Brown University undergraduate research assistants, Drew Hawkinson and Alan Mendoza, for insights on the they/them/their movement on campus. Laura Kipnis explains, "Sex on campus isn't just confusing. It's schizophrenic" (2017, 36).

4. Muguet 2017.

5. Spade 2015 [2011], 209; Foucault 1980, xiii.

6. Halberstam 2018, 9.

7. See Núñez Noriega 2014.

8. In 2012, Argentina passed a comprehensive transgender rights law allowing anyone to fill out a form, without approval of a judge or a doctor, to change their legal gender identity. In December 2018, Germany's highest court ruled that binary gender designations were discriminatory and that, with medical authorization, Germans could choose "diverse" on birth certificates and other legal records. LGBTQ groups objected that no medical approval should be required. See Eddy 2018.

9. Luhrmann 2000, 8. She was writing in a different context (the medical training of psychiatry students), but her point is germane here, too.

10. Bruni 2018. His conservative colleague David Brooks wrote around this same time, "I disagree with academic feminism a lot—with those vague oppressor stories about the patriarchy, with the strange unwillingness to admit inherited-gender differences and with the tone of faculty lounge militancy" (Brooks 2018). Those inherited-gender differences are

left unspecified, naturally, because such allegations need no explanation or justification if we take them for granted.

11. Dallek 2004, 315.

12. Nussbaum 2018.

13. Wang 2013, 12; Gould 1978, 532.

14. Bannon and Correia 2006, 5.

15. On alpha and beta male baboons, for example, see Gesquiere et al. 2011, 357.

16. Sahlins 1976, 101. Similarly, although Karl Marx was an early and devoted fan of Darwin's work, he wrote a letter to Friedrich Engels on June 18, 1862, in which he ruminated on certain problems in the naturalist's latest revelations:

> I'm amused that Darwin, at whom I've been taking another look, should say that he also applies the "Malthusian" theory to plants and animals, as though in Mr. Malthus's case the whole thing didn't lie in its not being applied to plants and animals, but only—with its geometric progression—to humans as against plants and animals. It is remarkable how Darwin rediscovers, among the beasts and plants, the society of England with its division of labor, competition, opening up of new markets, "inventions" and Malthusian "struggle for existence." It is Hobbes' *bellum omnium contra omnes* [the war of all against all] and is reminiscent of Hegel's *Phenomenology*, in which civil society figures as an "intellectual animal kingdom," whereas, in Darwin, the animal kingdom figures in civil society.

17. Fausto-Sterling 1992, 160. Agustín Fuentes writes: "If we believe we are aggressive at our base, that males stripped of social constraints will resort to a brutish nature, then we will expect and accept certain types of violence as inevitable. This means that instead of really trying to understand and rectify the horrific and complex realities of rape, genocide, civil war, and torture, we will chalk at least a part of these events up to human nature" (2012, 154).

18. Sherry Ortner asked, "Is female to male as nature is to culture?" (1972, 5).

19. For example, McCormack and Strathern 1980.

20. Ortner 1996, 176.

21. Donald J. Trump, as quoted in Scott 2018.

22. See the English translation in Paredes 1993 [1967]. My thanks to Sherry Ortner for this example, offered in response to a lecture I gave at UCLA that included my thoughts about her earlier nature-culture comparison.

BIBLIOGRAPHY

Ahmed, S. Faisal, and Martina Rodie. 2010. "Investigation and Initial Management of Ambiguous Genitalia." *Best Practice and Research Clinical Endocrinology and Metabolism* 24 (2): 197–218.

Albee, Edward. 2000. *The Goat, or, Who Is Sylvia?* New York: Overlook Press.

Appiah, Kwame Anthony. 2018. *The Ties That Bind: Rethinking Identity.* New York: Liveright.

Archer, John. 2006. "Testosterone and Human Aggression: An Evaluation of the Challenge Hypothesis." *Neuroscience and Biobehavioral Reviews* 30 (3): 319–345.

Aristophanes. 1994 [411 BC]. *Lysistrata*. New York: Grove.

Arizpe, Lourdes. 1990. "Foreword: Democracy for a Small Two-Gender Planet." In *Women and Social Change in Latin America*, edited by Elizabeth Jelin, xiv–xx. London: Zed.

Austen, Ian. 2016. "Women in Canadian Military Report Widespread Sexual Assault." *New York Times*, November 29, 2016.

Awori, Thelma, Catherine Lutz, and Paban J. Thapa. 2013. "Expert Mission to Evaluate Risks to SEA Prevention Efforts in MINUSTAH, UNMIL, MONUSCO, and UNMISS." static1.squarespace.com/static/514a0127 e4b04d7440e8045d/t/55afcfa1e4b07b89d11d35ae/1437585313823 /2013+Expert+Team+Report+FINAL.pdf.

Bannon, Ian, and Maria C. Correia. 2006. *The Other Half of Gender: Men's Issues in Development*. Washington, DC: International Bank for Reconstruction and Development, World Bank.

Barash, David. 1980. *Sociobiology: The Whisperings Within*. London: Souvenir.

Barlow, Tani E. 2004. *The Question of Women in Chinese Feminism*. Durham, NC: Duke University Press.

Bartra, Roger. 2014. *The Anthropology of the Brain: Consciousness, Culture, and Free Will*. Cambridge: Cambridge University Press.

Bekiempis, Victoria. 2015. "When Campus Rapists Don't Think They're Rapists." *Newsweek*, January 9, 2015.

Bender, Marylin. 1970. "Doctors Deny Woman's Hormones Affect Her As an Executive." *New York Times*, July 31, 1970.

Berger, John. 2009. *Why Look at Animals?* London: Penguin.

Bernstein, Jacob. 2017. "Is There Anything Ansel Elgort Can't Do?" *New York Times*, July 1, 2017.

Birenbaum-Carmeli, Daphna, Yana Diamand, and Maram Abu Yaman. 2015. "On Fatherhood in a Conflict Zone: Gaza Fathers and Their Children's Cancer Treatments." In *Globalized Fatherhood*, edited by Marcia C. Inhorn, Wendy Chavkin, and José-Alberto Navarro, 152–174. New York: Berghahn.

Blow, Charles M. 2017. "Trump Mauls the Language." *New York Times*, July 17, 2017.

Bourke, Joanna. 2007. *Rape: Sex, Violence, History*. London: Virago.

Brandes, Stanley. 1980. *Metaphors of Masculinity: Sex and Status in Andalusian Folklore*. Philadelphia: University of Pennsylvania Press.

———. 2002. *Staying Sober in Mexico City*. Austin: University of Texas Press.

Bribiescas, Richard G. 2006. *Men: Evolutionary and Life-History*. Cambridge, MA: Harvard University Press.

Bribiescas, Richard G., Peter T. Ellison, and Peter B. Gray. 2012. "Male Life History, Reproductive Effort, and the Evolution of the Genus *Homo*: New Directions and Perspectives." Supplement, *Current Anthropology* 53 (6): S424–S435.

Brooks, David. 2018. "Two Cheers for Feminism!" *New York Times*, October 12, 2018.

Brown, Wendy. 2006. *Regulating Aversion: Tolerance in the Age of Identity and Empire*. Princeton, NJ: Princeton University Press.

———. 2014. *Walled States, Waning Sovereignty*. New York: Zone.

Brownell, Susan, and Jeffrey Wasserstrom, eds. 2002. *Chinese Femininities / Chinese Masculinities*. Berkeley: University of California Press.

Brubaker, Rogers. 2016. *Trans: Gender and Race in an Age of Unsettled Identities*. Princeton, NJ: Princeton University Press.

Bruni, Frank. 2016. "Hillary's Male Tormentors." *New York Times*, November 2, 2016.

————. 2018. "The Many Faces of Brett Kavanaugh." *New York Times*, September 25, 2018.

Burke, James Lee. 2016. *The Jealous Kind*. New York: Simon and Schuster.

Campbell, Benjamin, Paul Leslie, and Kenneth Campbell. 2006. "Age-Related Changes in Testosterone and SHGB [sex hormone binding globulin] Among Turkana Males." *American Journal of Human Biology* 18 (1): 71–82.

Clausewitz, Carl von. 1989 [1832]. *On War*. Princeton, NJ: Princeton University Press.

Collins, Randall. 2008. *Violence: A Micro-sociological Theory*. Princeton, NJ: Princeton University Press.

Connell, Raewyn [Robert Connell]. 2000. "Arms and the Man: Using the New Research on Masculinity to Understand Violence and Promote Peace in the Contemporary World." In *Male Roles, Masculinities and Violence: A Culture of Peace Perspective*, edited by Ingeborg Breines, Robert Connell, and Ingrid Eide, 21–33. Paris: UNESCO.

Cooper, Alexia, and Erica L. Smith. 2011. "Homicide Trends in the United States, 1980–2008." Washington, DC: Bureau of Justice Statistics, Office of Justice Programs, US Department of Justice.

Culp-Ressler, Tara. 2015. "1 in 3 College Men in Survey Say They Would Rape a Woman if They Could Get Away with It." *Think Progress*, January 11, 2015. thinkprogress.org/1-in-3-college-men-in-survey-say-they -would-rape-a-woman-if-they-could-get-away-with-it-ffa7406b9778.

Dallek, Robert. 2004. *Flawed Giant: Lyndon Johnson and His Times, 1961–1973*. Oxford: Oxford University Press.

Darwin, Charles. 2009 [1872]. *The Expression of Emotion in Man and Animals*. New York: Penguin.

Davies, Julian. 2010. "Anthropomorphism in Science." *European Molecular Biology Organization* 11 (10): 721.

Davis, Deborah. 2010. "Who Gets the House? Re-negotiating Property Rights in Post-socialist Urban China." *Modern China* 36 (5): 463–492.

Davis, Deborah, and Sara Friedman, eds. 2014. *Wives, Husbands, Lovers: Marriage and Sexuality in Hong Kong, Taiwan, and Urban China*. Stanford, CA: Stanford University Press.

Davis, Natalie Zemon. 1983. *The Return of Martin Guerre*. Cambridge, MA: Harvard University Press.

Dawkins, Richard. 1976. *The Selfish Gene*. Oxford: Oxford University Press.

de Beauvoir, Simone. 1970 [1949]. *The Second Sex*. New York: Bantam.

Derrida, Jacques. 2002. "The Animal That Therefore I Am (More to Follow)." *Critical Inquiry* 28 (2): 369–418.

de Waal, Frans. 1999. "Anthropomorphism and Anthropodenial: Consistency in Our Thinking About Humans and Other Animals." *Philosophical Topics* 27 (1): 255–280.

———. 2001. *The Ape and the Sushi Master: Cultural Reflections of a Primatologist*. New York: Basic Books.

———. 2013. *The Bonobo and the Atheist: In Search of Humanism Among the Primates*. New York: W. W. Norton.

———. 2016. *Are We Smart Enough to Know How Smart Animals Are?* New York: W. W. Norton.

Diamond, Jared. 1999. *Guns, Germs, and Steel: The Fates of Human Societies*. New York: W. W. Norton.

Doi, Hirokazu, Ilaria Basadonne, Paola Venuti, and Kazuyuki Shinohara. 2018. "Negative Correlation Between Salivary Testosterone Concentration and Preference for Sophisticated Music in Males." *Personality and Individual Differences* 125: 106–111.

Domhoff, G. William. 1975. *Bohemian Grove and Other Retreats: A Study in Ruling-Class Cohesiveness*. New York: HarperCollins.

Dovy, Dana. 2018. "Men Who Like Jazz Have Less Testosterone Than Those Who Like Rock." *Newsweek*, January 19, 2018.

Downs, Laura L. 2002. "PMS, Psychosis and Culpability: Sound or Misguided Defense?" *Journal of Forensic Science* 47 (5): 1–7.

Duden, Barbara, and Silja Samerski. 2007. "'Pop Genes': An Investigation of 'the Gene' in Popular Parlance." In *Biomedicine as Culture: Instrumental Practices, Technoscientific Knowledge, and New Modes of Life*, edited by Regula Valérie Burri and Joseph Dumit, 167–189. New York: Routledge.

Dyble, M., G. D. Salali, N. Chaudhary, A. Page, D. Smith, J. Thompson, L. Vinicius, R. Mace, and A. B. Migliano. 2015. "Sex Equality Can Explain the Unique Social Structure of Hunter-Gatherer Bands." *Science* 348 (6236): 796–798.

Eddy, Melissa. 2018. "Not Male or Female? Germans Can Now Choose 'Diverse.'" *New York Times*, December 14, 2018.

Edwards, Sarah R., Kathryn A. Bradshaw, and Verlin B. Hinsz. 2014. "Denying Rape but Endorsing Forceful Intercourse: Exploring Differences Among Responders." *Violence and Gender* 1 (4): 188–193.

Eliot, Lise. 2009. *Pink Brain, Blue Brain: How Small Differences Grow into Troublesome Gaps—and What We Can Do About It*. New York: Houghton Mifflin.

Farquhar, Judith. 2002. *Appetites: Food and Sex in Post-Socialist China*. Durham, NC: Duke University Press.

Fausto-Sterling, Anne. 1992. *Myths of Gender: Biological Theories About Women and Men*, rev. ed. New York: Basic Books.

———. 2000. *Sexing the Body: Gender Politics and the Construction of Sexuality*. New York: Basic.

Fausto-Sterling, Anne, David Crews, Jihyun Sung, Cynthia García-Coll, and Ronald Seifer. 2015. "Multimodal Sex-Related Differences in Infant and in Infant-Directed Maternal Behaviors During Months Three Through Twelve of Development." *Developmental Psychology* 51 (10): 1351–1366.

Filipovic, Jill. 2015. " Study: 1 in 3 Men Would Rape If They Wouldn't Get Caught or Face Consequences." *Cosmopolitan*, January 12, 2015.

Fine, Cordelia. 2017. *Testosterone Rex: Myths of Sex, Science, and Society*. New York: W. W. Norton.

Fink, Sheri. 2017. "Las Vegas Gunman's Brain Will Be Scrutinized for Clues to the Killing." *New York Times*, October 26, 2017.

Finnström, Verker. 2008. *Living with Bad Surroundings: War, History, and Everyday Moments in Northern Uganda*. Durham, NC: Duke University Press.

Fisher, William A., and Donn Byrne. 1978. "Differences in Response to Erotica: Love Versus Lust." *Journal of Personality and Social Psychology* 36 (2): 117–125.

Foucault, Michel. 1980. *Herculine Barbin: Being the Recently Discovered Memoirs of a Nineteenth Century French Hermaphrodite*, translated by Richard McDougall. New York: Vintage.

Freud, Sigmund. 1990 [1913]. *Totem and Taboo*. New York: W. W. Norton.

———. 1995 [1918]. "From the History of an Infantile Neurosis ('Wolf Man')." In *The Freud Reader*, edited by Peter Gay, 400–426. New York: W. W. Norton.

Fuentes, Augustín. 2012. *Race, Monogamy, and Other Lies They Told You: Busting Myths About Human Nature*. Berkeley: University of California Press.

Galanes, Philip. 2018. "The Mind Meld of Bill Gates and Steven Pinker." *New York Times*, January 27, 2018.

Gesquiere, Laurence R., Niki H. Learn, M. Carolina M. Simao, Patrick O. Onyango, Susan C. Alberts, and Jeanne Altmann. 2011. "Life at the Top: Rank and Stress in Wild Male Baboons." *Science* 333 (6040): 357–360.

Global Industry Analysts, Inc. 2018. "Testosterone Replacement Therapy (TRT) — Market Analysis, Trends, and Forecasts by Global Industry Analysts, Inc., February 2018." www.strategyr.com/market-report-testosterone -replacement-therapy-trt-forecasts-global-industry-analysts-inc.asp.

Gordon, Deborah M. 2010. *Ant Encounters: Interaction Networks and Colony Behavior*. Princeton, NJ: Princeton University Press.

Gould, Stephen J. 1978. "Sociobiology: The Art of Storytelling." *New Scientist* 80 (1129): 530–533.

———. 1995. "Ordering Nature by Budding and Full-Breasted Sexuality." In *Dinosaur in a Haystack: Reflections in Natural History*, 427–441. New York: Harmony Books.

Gowaty, Patty A. 2010. "Forced or Aggressively Coerced Copulation." In *Encyclopedia of Animal Behavior*, edited by Michael D. Breed and Janice Moore, 759–763. Burlington, MA: Elsevier.

Graeber, David. 2005. "Fetishism as Social Creativity, or, Fetishes Are Gods in the Process of Construction." *Anthropological Theory* 5 (4): 407–438.

Grossman, Dave. 2009. *On Killing: The Psychological Cost of Learning to Kill in War and Society*. New York: Back Bay Books.

Gutmann, Matthew. 2006 [1996]. *The Meanings of Macho: Being a Man in Mexico City*. Berkeley: University of California Press.

———. 1999. "Ethnicity, Alcohol, and Acculturation." *Social Science & Medicine* 48 (2): 173–184.

———. 2002. *The Romance of Democracy: Compliant Defiance in Mexico City*. Berkeley: University of California Press.

———. 2007. *Fixing Men: Sex, Birth Control, and AIDS in Mexico*. Berkeley: University of California Press.

Gutmann, Matthew, and Catherine Lutz. 2010. *Breaking Ranks: Iraq Veterans Speak Out Against the War*. Berkeley: University of California Press.

Gwatkin, Davidson R. 1979. "Political Will and Family Planning: The Implications of India's Emergency Experience." *Population and Development Review* 5 (1): 29–59.

Halberstam, Jack. 2018. *Trans*: A Quick and Quirky Account of Gender Variability*. Berkeley: University of California Press.

Hamer, Dean, and Peter Copeland. 1994. *The Science of Desire: The Search for the Gay Gene and the Biology of Behavior*. New York: Simon and Schuster.

Harrington, Anne. 2019. *Mind Fixers: Psychiatry's Troubled Search for the Biology of Mental Illness*. New York: W. W. Norton.

Heald, Susan. 1999. *Manhood and Morality: Sex, Violence and Ritual in Gisu Society*. New York: Routledge.

Heider, Karl. 1976. "Dani Sexuality: A Low Energy System." *Man* 11 (2): 188–201.

Herbert, Joe. 2015. *Testosterone: Sex, Power, and the Will to Win*. Oxford: Oxford University Press.

Herdt, Gilbert. 1994. *Guardians of the Flutes: Idioms of Masculinity*. Chicago: University of Chicago Press.

Hershatter, Gail. 1996. "Sexing Modern China." In *Remapping China: Fissures in Historical Terrain*, edited by Gail Hershatter, Emily Honig, Jonathan N. Lipman, and Randall Stross, 77–93. Stanford, CA: Stanford University Press.

Hirsch, Jennifer. 2003. *A Courtship After Marriage: Sexuality and Love in Mexican Transnational Families*. Berkeley: University of California Press.

Hirsch, Jennifer, and Constance Nathanson. 2001. "Some Traditional Methods Are More Modern Than Others: Rhythm, Withdrawal and the Changing Meanings of Sexual Intimacy in the Mexican Companionate Marriage." *Culture, Health and Sexuality* 3 (4): 413–428.

Hoberman, John. 2005. *Testosterone Dreams: Rejuvenation, Aphrodisia, Doping*. Berkeley: University of California Press.

Hochschild, Arlie, with Anne Machung. 1989. *The Second Shift: Working Parents and the Revolution at Home*. New York: Viking.

Hofstadter, Richard. 1992 [1944]. *Social Darwinism in American Thought*. Boston: Beacon Press.

Hönekopp, Johannes, and Steven Watson. 2011. "Meta-analysis of the Relationship Between Digit-Ratio 2D:4D and Aggression." *Personality and Individual Differences* 51: 381–386.

Hong Fincher, Leta. 2014. *Leftover Women: The Resurgence of Gender Inequality in China*. New York: Zed.

Hrdy, Sarah Blaffer. 1981. *The Woman That Never Evolved*. Cambridge, MA: Harvard University Press.

———. 2000. "The Optimal Number of Fathers: Evolution, Demography and History in the Shaping of Female Mate Preferences." *Annals of the New York Academy of Sciences* 907 (1): 75–96.

———. 2009. *Mothers and Others: The Evolutionary Origins of Mutual Understanding*. Cambridge, MA: Harvard University Press.

Huerta Rojas, Fernando. 1999. *El juego del hombre: Deporte y masculinidad entre obreros de Volkswagen*. Mexico City: Plaza y Valdés.

Hurston, Zora Neale. 2006 [1937]. *Their Eyes Were Watching God*. New York: Harper.

Hyde, Janet Shibley. 2005. "The Gender Similarities Hypothesis." *American Psychologist* 60 (6): 581–592.

Isaacson, Walter. 2017. "Resistance Is Futile." *New York Times Book Review*, June 25, 2017.

Joel, Daphna. 2011. "Male or Female? Brains Are Intersex." *Frontiers in Integrative Neuroscience* 5: 1–5.

———. 2016. "Captured in Terminology: Sex, Sex Categories, and Sex Differences." *Feminism and Psychology* 26 (3): 335–345.

Johnson, Ian. 2014. "Sex in China: An Interview with Li Yinhe." *New York Review of Books*, September 9, 2014.

Jordan-Young, Rebecca M. 2010. *Brain Storm: The Flaws in the Science of Sex Differences*. Cambridge, MA: Harvard University Press.

Kafka, Franz. 2013 [1917]. *A Report for an Academy*. CreateSpace.

Kan, Karoline. 2017. "China, Where the Pressure to Marry Is Strong, and the Advice Flows Online." *New York Times*, June 18, 2017.

Keller, Evelyn Fox. 2010. *The Mirage of a Space Between Nature and Nurture*. Durham, NC: Duke University Press.

Kimmel, Michael. 1994. "Masculinity as Homophobia: Fear, Shame and Silence in the Construction of Gender Identity." In *Theorizing Masculinities*, edited by Harry Brod and Michael Kaufman, 119–141. Newbury Park, CA: Sage.

———. 2003. "An Unnatural History of Rape." In *Evolution, Gender, and Rape*, edited by Cheryl Brown Travis, 221–233. Cambridge, MA: MIT Press.

Kingkade, Tyler. 2015. "Nearly One-Third of College Men in Study Say They Would Commit Rape." *Huffington Post*, January 9, 2015.

Kipnis, Laura. 2014. *Men: Notes from an Ongoing Investigation*. New York: Picador.

———. 2017. *Unwanted Advances: Sexual Paranoia Comes to Campus*. New York: HarperCollins.

Kogan, Terry S. 2010. "Sex Separation: The Cure-All for Victorian Social Anxiety." In *Toilet: Public Restrooms and the Politics of Sharing*, edited by Harvey Molotch and Laura Norén, 145–164. New York: New York University Press.

Kolata, Gina. 2012. "Seeing Answers in Genome of Gunman." *New York Times*, December 24, 2012.

Krugman, Paul. 1997. "Biobabble." *Slate*, October 24, 1997.

Kruttschnitt, Candace. 2013. "Gender and Crime." *Annual Review of Sociology* 39: 291–308.

Lam, Theodora, and Brenda S. A. Yeoh. 2015. "Long-Distance Fathers, Left-Behind Fathers, and Returnee Fathers: Changing Fathering Practices in Indonesia and the Philippines." In *Globalized Fatherhood*, edited by Marcia C. Inhorn, Wendy Chavkin, and José-Alberto Navarro, 103–125. New York: Berghahn.

Lancaster, Roger. 2003. *The Trouble with Nature: Sex in Science and Popular Culture*. Berkeley: University of California Press.

Laqueur, Thomas. 1990. *Making Sex: Body and Gender from the Greeks to Freud*. Cambridge, MA: Harvard University Press.

———. 2002. "Foreword." In *Chinese Femininities / Chinese Masculinities: A Reader*, edited by Susan Brownell and Jeffrey Wasserstrom, xi–xiv. Berkeley: University of California Press.

Leach, Edmund R. 1964. "Anthropological Aspects of Language: Animal Categories and Verbal Abuse." In *New Directions in the Study of Language*, edited by E. H. Lenneberg, 23–63. Cambridge, MA: MIT Press.

Lee, Spike. 2015. *Chi-Raq*. Amazon Studios.

Lévi-Strauss, Claude. 1971 [1963]. *Totemism*. Boston, MA: Beacon.

Lewis, James W. 1990. "Premenstrual Syndrome as a Criminal Defense." *Archives of Sexual Behavior* 19 (5): 425–441.

Lewis, Oscar. 1963. *Life in a Mexican Village: Tepoztlán Restudied*. Urbana: University of Illinois Press.

Lock, Margaret. 2012. "From Genetics to Postgenomics and the Discovery of the New Social Body." In *Medical Anthropology at the Intersections: Histories, Activisms, and Futures*, edited by Marcia C. Inhorn and Emily A. Wentzell, 129–160. Durham, NC: Duke University Press.

———. 2013. "The Epigenome and Nature/Nurture Reunification: A Challenge for Anthropology." *Medical Anthropology* 32 (4): 291–308.

———. 2015. "Comprehending the Body in the Era of the Epigenome." *Current Anthropology* 56 (2): 151–177.

———. 2018. "Mutable Environments and Permeable Human Bodies." *Journal of the Royal Anthropological Institute* 24: 449–474.

Lock, Margaret, and Gisli Palsson. 2016. *Can Science Resolve the Nature/Nurture Debate?* Cambridge, UK: Polity Press.

Lodge, David. 2001. *Thinks . . . .* New York: Penguin.

Louie, Kam. 2002. *Theorising Chinese Masculinity: Society and Gender in China*. Cambridge: Cambridge University Press.

———, ed. 2016. *Changing Chinese Masculinities: From Imperial Pillars of State to Global Real Men*. Hong Kong: Hong Kong University Press.

Luhrmann, T. M. 2000. *Of Two Minds: An Anthropologist Looks at American Psychiatry*. New York: Vintage.

Luo Yuan. 2010. «伪娘太多的中国是危险的» (It's dangerous to have too many feminine men in China). 环球时报 (*Global Times*). April 11, 2010, 1.

Lutz, Catherine, ed. 2009. *The Bases of Empire: The Global Struggle Against US Military Posts*. New York: New York University Press.

Lu Xun. 1990 [1918]. "Diary of a Madman." *Diary of a Madman and Other Stories*, translated by William A. Lyell. Honolulu: University of Hawaii Press.

Malamuth, Neil M. 1996. "Sexually Explicit Media, Gender Differences, and Evolutionary Theory." *Journal of Communication* 46 (3): 8–31.

"Many US College Men Deny Rape but Endorse Forceful Intercourse." 2015. *Financial Express*, January 13, 2015. https://www.financialexpress.com/india-news/many-us-college-men-deny-rape-but-endorse-forceful-intercourse/29581.

Marks, Jonathan. 2002. *What It Means to Be 98% Chimpanzee: Apes, People, and Their Genes*. Berkeley: University of California Press.

———. 2015. *Tales of the Ex-Apes: How We Think About Human Evolution*. Oakland: University of California Press.

Martin, Emily. 1994. "The Ethnography of Natural Selection in the 1990s." *Cultural Anthropology* 9 (3): 383–397.

———. 2003. "What Is 'Rape'?—Toward a Historical, Ethnographic Approach." In *Evolution, Gender, and Rape*, edited by Cheryl Brown Travis, 363–381. Cambridge, MA: MIT Press.

Marx, Karl. 1977 [1844]. *Critique of Hegel's Philosophy of Right*. Cambridge: Cambridge University Press.

———. 1980 [1862]. "Letter to Friedrich Engels on 18 June." In *Letters, 1860–64*. Vol. 41 in *Marx/Engels Collected Works*, 380. London: Lawrence and Wishart.

McCormack, Carol, and Marilyn Strathern. 1980. *Nature, Culture, and Gender*. Cambridge: Cambridge University Press.

McNamara, Robert. 1974. "The World Bank Perspective on Population Growth." In *Dynamics of Population Policy in Latin America*, edited by Terry L. McCoy, 107–121. Cambridge, MA: Ballinger.

Mead, Margaret. 2001 [1928]. *Coming of Age in Samoa*. New York: William Morrow.

Mernissi, Fatima. 1987. *Beyond the Veil: Male-Female Dynamics in a Muslim Society*. Bloomington: Indiana University Press.

Merriman, Mazie Katherine. 2015. "China's 'Leftover' Women Phenomenon: Media Portrayal and 'Leftover' Voices." BA thesis, International Studies, University of Mississippi.

Miano Borruso, Marinella. 2002. *Hombre, mujer y muxe' en el Istmo de Tehuantepec*. Mexico City: Plaza y Valdés, CONACULTA-INAH.

Milam, Erika Lorraine. 2019. *Creatures of Cain: The Hunt for Human Nature in Cold War America*. Princeton, NJ: Princeton University Press.

Mistry, Rohinton. 1997. *A Fine Balance*. New York: Vintage.

Molotch, Harvey, and Laura Norén, eds. 2010. *Toilet: Public Restrooms and the Politics of Sharing*. New York: New York University Press.

Monsiváis, Carlos. 1988. *Escenas de pudor y liviandad*. Mexico City: Grijalbo.

———. 1997. *Mexican Postcards*, translated by John Kraniauskas. London: Verso.

Morgentaler, Abraham. 2009. *Testosterone for Life: Recharge Your Vitality, Sex Drive, Muscle Mass & Overall Health!* New York: McGraw Hill.

Muguet, Julien. 2017. "Edouard Philippe décide de bannir l'écriture inclusive des textes officiels." *Le Monde*, November 21, 2017.

Nagel, Thomas. 1974. "What Is It Like to Be a Bat?" *Philosophical Review* 83 (4): 435–450.

Núñez Noriega, Guillermo. 2014. *Just Between Us: An Ethnography of Male Identity and Intimacy in Rural Communities of Northern Mexico*. Tucson: University of Arizona Press.

Nussbaum, Martha. 2018. "The Roots of Male Rage, on Show at the Kavanaugh Hearing." *Washington Post*, September 29, 2018.

Oates, Joyce Carol. 1988. "Against Nature." In *(Woman) Writer: Occasions and Opportunities*. New York: E. P. Dutton.

Ortner, Sherry B. 1972. "Is Female to Male As Nature Is to Culture?" *Feminist Studies* 1 (2): 5–31.

———. 1996. "So, *Is* Female to Male As Nature Is to Culture?" In *Making Gender: The Politics and Erotics of Culture*, 172–180. Boston, MA: Beacon.

Oudshoorn, Nelly. 1994. *Beyond the Natural Body: An Archaeology of Sex Hormones*. New York: Routledge.

————. 2003. *The Male Pill: A Biography of a Technology in the Making*. Durham, NC: Duke University Press.

Paredes, Américo. 1993 [1967]. "The United States, Mexico, and *Machismo.*" In *Folklore and Culture on the Texas-Mexican Border*, 215–234. Austin: University of Texas Press.

Parker, Kathleen. 2010. "Obama: Our First Female President." *Washington Post*, June 30, 2010.

Parker, Richard. 1998. *Beneath the Equator: Cultures of Desire, Male Homosexuality, and Emerging Gay Communities in Brazil*. New York: Routledge.

Parrini, Rodrigo. 2007. *Panópticos y Laberintos: Subjetivación, deseo y corporalidad en una cárcel dehombres*. Mexico City: El Colegio de México.

Parsons, Talcott, and Robert F. Bales. 1955. *Family, Socialization and Interaction Process*. New York: Free Press.

Paz, Octavio. 2012 [1949]. *The Labyrinth of Solitude*. New York: Grove.

Peterson, Jordan B. 2018. *12 Rules for Life: An Antidote to Chaos*. Toronto: Random House.

Pierson, David P. 2005. "'Hey, They're Just Like Us!': Representations of the Animal World in the Discovery Channel's Nature Programming." *Journal of Popular Culture* 38 (4): 698–712.

Pile, John M., and Mark A. Barone. 2009. "Demographics of Vasectomy— USA and International." *Urologic Clinics of North America* 36 (3): 295–305.

Pinker, Steven. 2002. *The Blank Slate: The Modern Denial of Human Nature*. New York: Penguin.

Press, Marc P. 1983. "Premenstrual Stress Syndrome as a Defense in Criminal Cases." *Duke Law Journal* 32 (1): 176–195.

Prum, Richard O. 2017. *The Evolution of Beauty: How Darwin's Forgotten Theory of Mate Choice Shapes the Animal World—And Us*. New York: Doubleday.

Raine, Adrian. 2013. *The Anatomy of Violence: The Biological Roots of Crime*. New York: Vintage.

Reddy, Gayatri. 2005. *With Respect to Sex: Negotiating Hijra Identity in South India*. Chicago: University of Chicago Press.

"Report of the Committee on the Unrecognized Single-Gender Social Organizations." 2017. Harvard College. s3.amazonaws.com/media.thecrimson .com/pdf/2017/07/12/1323575.pdf.

Rich, Adrienne. 1996. *Of Woman Born: Motherhood as Experience and Institution*. New York: W. W. Norton.

Richardson, Sarah S. 2013. *Sex Itself: The Search for Male and Female in the Human Genome*. Chicago, IL: University of Chicago Press.

———. 2017. "Plasticity and Programming: Feminism and the Epigenetic Imaginary." *Signs* 43 (1): 29–52.

Rubin, Gayle. 1984. "Thinking Sex: Notes for a Radical Theory of the Politics of Sexuality." In *Pleasure and Danger: Exploring Female Sexuality*, edited by Carole S. Vance, 3–44. New York: Routledge.

Sahlins, Marshall. 1976. *Use and Abuse of Biology: An Anthropological Critique of Sociobiology*. Ann Arbor: University of Michigan Press.

Sakai, Junko. 2003. *Makeinu no toboe* (The distant barking of losing dogs). Tokyo: Kundansha.

Sanday, Peggy Reeves. 1981. "The Socio-Cultural Context of Rape: A Cross-Cultural Study." *Journal of Social Issues* 37 (4): 5–27.

———. 2003. "Rape-Free Versus Rape-Prone: How Culture Makes a Difference." In *Evolution, Gender, and Rape*, edited by Cheryl Brown Travis, 337–361. Cambridge, MA: MIT Press.

Sandberg, Sheryl. 2013a. *Lean In: Women, Work, and the Will to Lead*. New York: Knopf.

———. 2013b. 向前一步：女性，工作及领导意志 (One step forward: Women, work, and the will to lead). Beijing: Zhongxin Publishing.

Sapolsky, Robert M. 1997. *The Trouble with Testosterone and Other Essays on the Biology of the Human Predicament*. New York: Simon and Schuster.

———. 2005. *Monkeyluv: And Other Essays on Our Lives as Animals*. New York: Scribner.

———. 2017. *Behave: The Biology of Humans at Our Best and Worst*. New York: Penguin.

Scheper-Hughes, Nancy, and Margaret M. Lock. 1987. "The Mindful Body: A Prolegomenon to Future Work in Medical Anthropology." *Medical Anthropology Quarterly* 1 (1): 6–41.

Scott, Eugene. 2018. "In Reference to 'Animals,' Trump Evokes an Ugly History of Dehumanization." *Washington Post*, May 16, 2018.

Shakespeare, William. 2004 [1608]. *King Lear*. New York: Simon and Schuster.

Smuts, Barbara. 1992. "Male Aggression Against Women: An Evolutionary Perspective." *Human Nature* 3 (1): 1–44.

Solomon, Lee. 1995. "Premenstrual Syndrome: The Debate Surrounding Criminal Defense." *Maryland Law Review* 54 (2): 571–600.

Sontag, Susan. 2002. "Looking at War: Photography's View of Devastation and Death." *New Yorker*, December 9, 2002.

Spade, Dean. 2015 [2011]. *Normal Life: Administrative Violence, Critical Trans Politics, and the Limits of Law*. Durham, NC: Duke University Press.

Stephen, Lynn. 2002. "Sexualities and Genders in Zapotec Oaxaca." *Latin American Perspectives* 29 (2): 41–59.

Taggart, James. 1992. "Gender Segregation and Cultural Constructions of Sexuality in Two Hispanic Societies." *American Ethnologist* 19 (1): 75–96.

Tarlo, Emma. 2003. *Unsettling Memories: Narratives of the Emergency in Delhi*. Berkeley: University of California Press.

Thao, Vu Thi. 2015. "When the Pillar of the Home Is Shaking: Female Labor Migration and Stay-at-Home Fathers in Vietnam." In *Globalized Fatherhood*, edited by Marcia C. Inhorn, Wendy Chavkin, and José-Alberto Navarro, 129–151. New York: Berghahn.

Thornhill, Randy, and Craig T. Palmer. 2000. *A Natural History of Rape: Biological Bases of Sexual Coercion*. Cambridge, MA: MIT Press.

Tiger, Lionel. 1984 [1969]. *Men in Groups*. New York: Marion Boyars.

"Transcript: Donald Trump's Taped Comments About Women." 2016. *New York Times*, October 8, 2016.

Travis, Cheryl Brown, ed. 2003. *Evolution, Gender, and Rape*. Cambridge, MA: MIT Press.

United Nations Office on Drugs and Crime. 2014. *Global Study on Homicide 2013: Trends/Contexts/Data*. Vienna: Research and Trend Analysis Branch, Division for Policy Analysis and Public Affairs, United Nations Office on Drugs and Crime.

Uretsky, Elanah. 2016. *Occupational Hazards: Sex, Business, and HIV in Post-Mao China*. Stanford, CA: Stanford University Press.

Vargas Llosa, Mario. 1978. *Captain Pantoja and the Special Service*. New York: Harper and Row.

Viveros, Mara. 2002. *De quebradores y de cumplidores: Sobre hombres, masculinidades y relaciones de género en Colombia*. Bogotá: Universidad Nacional de Colombia.

Von Drehle, David. 2014. "Manopause?! Aging, Insecurity and the $2 Billion Testosterone Industry." *Time*, July 31, 2014.

Wang, Lingzhen. 2013. "Gender and Sexual Differences in 1980s China: Introducing Li Xiaojiang." *Differences* 24 (2): 8–21.

Wang, Mengqi. 2018. "The 'Rigid Demand': The Culture of Home-Buying in Post-Socialist China." PhD diss., Anthropology, Brandeis University.

Wang, Pan. 2016. "Inventing Traditions: Television Dating Shows in the People's Republic of China." *Media, Culture, and Society* 39 (4): 504–519.

Waugh, Linda R. 1982. "Marked and Unmarked: A Choice Between Unequals in Semiotic Structure." *Semiotica* 38 (3/4): 299–318.

Wilson, Edward O. 2000 [1975]. *Sociobiology: The New Synthesis*. Cambridge, MA: Harvard University Press.

———. 2004 [1978]. *On Human Nature*. Cambridge, MA: Harvard University Press.

Winnicott, D. W. 1953. "Transitional Objects and Transitional Phenomena." *International Journal of Psycho-Analysis* 34 (2): 89–97.

Wolf, Larry L. 1975. "'Prostitution' Behavior in a Tropical Hummingbird." *Condor* 77 (2): 140–144.

Wolfe, Alexandra. 2014. "Weekend Confidential: E. O. Wilson—The Noted Biologist on Courting Controversy and the End of the Age of Man." *Wall Street Journal*, April 19, 2014.

Wong, Wang I., and Melissa Hines. 2016. "Interpreting Digit Ratio (2D:4D)—Behavior Correlations: 2D:4D Sex Difference, Stability, and Behavioral Correlates and Their Replicability in Young Children." *Hormones and Behavior* 78: 86–94.

Woolf, Virginia. 1938. *Three Guineas*. London: Hogarth Press.

Wrangham, Richard, and Dale Peterson. 1996. *Demonic Males: Apes and the Origins of Human Violence*. Boston: Houghton Mifflin.

Xi Jinping. 2012. 《习近平谈苏联解体》 (Xi Jinping discusses the disintegration of the Soviet Union). August 6, 2014, blog.sina.com.cn/s/blog _ae27d1f50102 uyrq.html.

Yang, Martin. 1945. *A Chinese Village: Taitou, Shantung Province*. New York: Columbia University Press.

Yang, Mayfair Mei-hui. 1999. "From Gender Erasure to Gender Difference: State Feminism, Consumer Sexuality, and Women's Public Sphere in China." In *Spaces of Their Own: Women's Public Sphere in Transnational China*, edited by Mayfair Mei-hui Yang, 35–67. Minneapolis: University of Minnesota Press.

Zeid Ra'ad Al Hussein. 2005. "A Comprehensive Strategy to Eliminate Future Sexual Exploitation and Abuse in United Nations Peacekeeping." New York: United Nations.

Zhang, Everett. 2015. *The Impotence Epidemic: Men's Medicine and Sexual Desire in Contemporary China*. Durham, NC: Duke University Press.

Zhang, Jun, and Peidong Sun. 2014. "When Are You Going to Get Married? Parental Matchmaking and Middle-Class Women in Contemporary Urban China." In *Wives, Husbands, and Lovers: Marriage and Sexuality in Hong Kong, Taiwan, and Urban China*, edited by Deborah S. Davis and Sara L. Friedman, 118–144. Stanford, CA: Stanford University Press.

Zheng, Tiantian. 2009a. *Ethnographies of Prostitution in Contemporary China*. New York: Palgrave.

———. 2009b. *Red Lights: The Lives of Sex Workers in Postsocialist China*. Minneapolis: University of Minnesota Press.

———. 2012. "Female Subjugation and Political Resistance." *Gender, Place and Culture* 19 (5): 652–669.

Zuk, Marlene. 2002. *Sexual Selections: What We Can and Can't Learn About Sex from Animals*. Berkeley: University of California Press.

INDEX

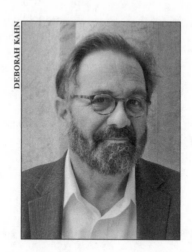

DEBORAH KAHN

MATTHEW GUTMANN is a professor of anthropology at Brown University who has spent thirty years exploring notions of masculinity across the United States, Latin America, and China. He has been a visiting professor at El Colegio de México and Nanjing University and is the author of eight books. He lives in Tiverton, Rhode Island.